SHAME AND THE SELF

Shame

AND THE

Self

◆ ◆ ◆ ◆

Francis J. Broucek

THE GUILFORD PRESS
New York   London

© 1991 The Guilford Press
A Division of Guilford Publications, Inc.
72 Spring Street, New York, NY 10012

Printed in the United States of America

This book is printed on acid-free paper.

Last digit is print number: 9 8 7 6 5 4 3 2 1

Library of Congress Cataloging-in-Publication Data

Broucek, Francis J.
  Shame and the Self / Francis J. Broucek.
    p.   cm.
  Includes bibliographical references and index.
  ISBN 0-89862-444-4
  1. Shame. 2. Self. 3. Psychology, Pathological. I. Title.
RC455.4.S53B76   1991
152.4—dc20   91-6797
                                                     CIP

For Peggy, Alison, Karen,
Margaret, and Eric

Foreword

When I was exploring the literature on shame for my first paper on the subject, I came upon a newly published article by Frank Broucek in the *International Journal of Psycho-Analysis*, "Shame and Its Relationship to Early Narcissistic Developments." In Broucek's work, I recognized that I had encountered an intellectual soulmate, a fellow traveler/shamenik who shared with me a perspective on the significance of shame to the self. After the shock wave eased, referring to the experience that follows the first reading of a work that seems to articulate most of the thoughts one is struggling to understand and put together about a given subject, I contacted Dr. Broucek to discuss his ideas, and to request a response to my paper on shame. Thus began an exchange over the years, which culminates now in my excitement at reading the current volume, and my pleasure and pride—a particular antonym of shame, as noted by Broucek—at being invited to write the Foreword.

Shame indeed remains central to narcissistic developments. And Broucek, to his credit, has included in this book the pivotal thoughts from his 1982 article about the *egotistical* (or grandiose, "idealized," haughty, and "unconflicted") and *dissociated* (or devalued, vulnerable) types of narcissist. Shame seems absent in the first, and "engulfing" in the second. To these types, he adds a new third, the *turbulent* type, who expresses "violent lability" between the manifest and dissociated types of narcissism. (I have referred to this lability as the "Dialectic of Narcissism" [Morrison, 1989].) Broucek further notes that shame may *instigate* the creation of egotistical narcissism as a defense against a sense of vulnerability, as well as the "splitting off" from awareness of grandiosity itself (analogous to Kohut's "vertical split").

This present volume takes Broucek's earlier thoughts about shame and narcissism and carries them into new realms (see Chapter 4, specifically) based as they are on intriguing conceptualizations about objective self-awareness. Here, he refers to the infant's evolving awareness, at about 18 months, of his condition as object in the eyes of others, leading to public awareness of the self, and self-awareness based on observation by the exterior 'other.' And with objective self-awareness comes the subjective experience of shame, a reflection of the "objectification" of the self (which Broucek refers to as a subject–OBJECT, or object alone). The constructs of objective self-awareness and objectification play major roles in Broucek's subsequent elaborations on shame.

Similarly, the distinction between the affect or feeling of shame, and the *sense of shame*, is an important addition to Broucek's former thinking. A *sense of shame* refers to "anticipatory shame," or "the discretionary function which makes us pause before saying or doing something which would arouse the painful feeling of shame in ourselves or another." Thus, the sense of shame serves as a "permanent safeguard of our psychic life." With attention to the sense of shame, then, Broucek anticipates his own, more gentle, lability between the pathological and the socially beneficial elements of shame that informs the rest of the book.

Building on these theoretical constructs, he turns to the clinical manifestations and applications of shame phenomena. Here, his unique and provocative qualities as a psychoanalytically-informed psychotherapist come to the fore. Often using his interest in shame as a background, he takes us into some controversial and unusual arenas and personal predilections, speaking to issues that he has clearly been mulling over for many years. I was fascinated to watch the author reveal himself as radically independent of and challenging to the psychoanalytic establishment, and at the same time, as a champion of some 'old-fashioned,' earthy values guided by the 'sense of shame' that he had elaborated upon in the theoretical section.

As a practicing psychoanalyst informed by the contributions of self-psychology, I was pleased to share Broucek's appreciation of the Kohutian perspective as a framework for understanding shame. In fact, his formulation of SUBJECT–object seems to have many elements in common with Kohut's 'self-object.' Broucek's independence of classical psychoanalysis is indicated by his suggestion that analysis itself often functions as a narcissistic enterprise (for both patient and analyst), and his related conceptualization of the role of transference in inducing shame, particularly for the patient, but potentially for the analyst as well. According to Broucek, the concept of transference implies an asymmetric relationship in which the patient becomes objectified, his feelings toward the analyst serving as the object of study rather than a source generating equivalent affective response from the analyst. Broucek believes that this mutually accepted 'arrangement' of patient objectification frequently induces shame.

These perspectives on the shame-inducing structure of psychotherapy itself, the transference in particular, and the narcissistic foundation of psychoanalysis are interesting observations, and clearly warn us of the dangers inherent in systematic 'perpetration' of rigid, experience-distant psychoanalytic interpretation and technique. His observations on the shame-inducing asymmetry of the analytic relationship, and on the analyst's lack of responsiveness to patients' expressions of desire in the transference, create helpful guidelines for attention to shame in treatment.

However, it seems to me that Broucek occasionally offers a reductionistic exposition of psychoanalysis, unmodified by more recent contributions to technique. For instance, emphasis on psychoanalysis as a two-person psychology (Modell, 1984) addresses the interactive quality of treatment that implies sensitivity to shame-induction. Similarly, Gill's (1984) attention to the here-and-now importance of the analyst in transference interaction, as well as Schwaber's (1983) focus on the analyst's contributions to transference feelings and 'psychic reality,' implicitly address the analytic potential for generation of shame. These recent additions to the theory of psychoanalytic technique should be considered as the reader follows Broucek's stimulating analysis of shame-induction and objectification in his clinical examples and discussion.

In the last section of his book, Broucek offers some surprises. In the chapter "Shame and Sexuality," he takes us back in time to a period when an interpersonal, intimate, and tender view of sex predominated, in which love and attachment to the object were viewed as an integral part of sexuality. Essentially, he suggests that the separation of sex as drive from sex as sensual attachment to the beloved object began with Freud, and has been elaborated into narcissistic, objectified states of pornography and sex-as-commerce, which are so prominent today. From Broucek's perspective, anticipated shame (at the separation of sexuality from the loved object) protects against the isolation of autoerotic sex that seems to prevail in contemporary society. Fundamentally, he presents a case for a sense of shame that will safeguard the self and support true intimacy and love—sexual and otherwise. This viewpoint relates again to Kohut's thinking—in this case, the Kohutian notion of autoerotic sex as a disintegration product of a self striving to preserve some quality of cohesion. On the other hand, Broucek's implicit emphasis on object love differs from Kohut's view on a separate developmental line for narcissism.

Finally, Broucek takes us on a fascinating journey through the ramifications of objectification, initiated by a bone-chilling, detailed interview with the 'exotic dancer' Olympia, who asserts right off "I am totally without shame." According to Broucek, the major instrument of contemporary objectification is the camera. He goes on to illustrate the intrusive, shame-inducing elements of the 'image' as perpetrated by that instrument. This attention to imaging also includes current medical emphasis on various 'scans' and 'resonances,' which play a part in the psychiatric importance placed on the (objectified) brain and its various 'visualizations.'

Reading *Shame and the Self* acquainted me with the latest thinking of an esteemed colleague and fellow toiler in the field of shame. As always, Frank Broucek brings a probing illumination to his investigation, as he sheds light on this most visual of the affects. It's fun to follow the turns of his mind, to accompany him on the journey that shame promotes. As always, Broucek is a skilled, compassionate clinician; but more, someone who can lead the subject of shame to a 'Jungian' turn, then a dip into the philosophical roots of psychology, then again a move into the mystical or the religious underpinnings of Christianity. No matter what the approach to shame, though, he is guided by a dedicated humanism that somehow manages to lift the study of shame from its potential burdensome heaviness into an uplifting optimism.

Move on, then, from this Foreword into what will be for you, the reader, an interesting, provocative, and (paradoxically) enjoyable study of shame.

ANDREW P. MORRISON
Boston Psychoanalytic Society and Institute
and Harvard Medical School

REFERENCES

Broucek, F. (1982). Shame and its relationship to early narcissistic developments. *International Journal of Psycho-Analysis*, 63, 369–378.

Gill, M. (1984). Psychoanalysis and psychotherapy: A revision. *International Review of Psycho-Analysis*, 11, 161–180.

Modell, A. (1984). *Psychoanalysis in a new context*. New York: International University Press.

Morrison, A. (1989). *Shame: The underside of narcissism*. Hillsdale, NJ: The Analytic Press.

Schwaber, E. (1983). Psychoanalytic listening and psychic reality. *International Journal of Psycho-Analysis*, 10, 379–392.

Preface

The psychoanalyst D. W. Winnicott said something to the effect that much clinical writing was autobiographical and represented an attempt to complete (or at least extend) the writer's analysis. I would certainly include the present work in that category, although I hope it is more than simply an extension of self-analysis. "Art begins in a wound . . ." says John Gardner (1978), and he goes on to say

> What we mean by "wound" in this case of course is some wound to personality and self-confidence, something that attacks or threatens the dignity and self-respect of the artist and must be overcome if his personality is to be healthy. The wound may take any number of forms: doubt about one's parentage, fear that one is a fool or freak, the crippling effect of psychological trauma or the potentially crippling effect of alienation from the society in which one feels at home, whether or not any such society really exists outside the fantasy of the artist. (p. 181)

It seems to me that Gardner's "wound" is anything that produces a heavy burden of shame for the artist and, as Gardner suggests, the artist's creativity stems from an attempt to heal that wound. I would extend Gardner's observations to include not only artists but many people who are engaged in creative work. The present work grew out of my own woundedness and gained added impetus through my gradually increasing awareness of a widespread human woundedness, shame based, which was most clearly evident in the hospitals, clinics, and consulting rooms where I spend my working life.

In developing my ideas about shame I have benefited enormously from the opportunity to share observations and exchange ideas with several respected colleagues who have made important contributions to the recent literature on shame. Donald Nathanson and I agreed and disagreed about various issues, but our lengthy telephone conversations (he lives in Philadelphia, I live in Kansas City) were always stimulating and helpful to me in clarifying certain aspects of the complicated nature of shame phenomena. I am also grateful to Andrew Morrison, who cheerfully agreed to write the foreword for this work. Morrison's work on shame and narcissism and my own fit rather closely together in most respects. Because of that our exchanges over the years have been very friendly and mutually supportive. My debt to Silvan Tomkins is also considerable. He generously spent a great many hours educating me on the subtleties of his affect theory, and our talks often included many in-depth discussions about shame.

Seymour Weingarten and his editorial staff at The Guilford Press deserve considerable credit for their efforts to give greater coherence and better form to my manuscript. Also my thanks to the anonymous reviewer who made many valuable suggestions for improving the overall organization of the book.

Special thanks and appreciation are owed to my wife, Peggy, who has endured the strains and sacrifices that accompany an undertaking such as this one, which consumed countless evenings and weekends. In addition to her patience and support she offered many valuable suggestions on stylistic matters and enriched the content of the work by bringing to my attention various materials from diverse sources relevant to my subject. Thanks also to my daughter Margaret who read earlier drafts of various chapters and with her writer's eye for syntactical and grammatical atrocities helped me produce a more lucid manuscript.

Appreciation is expressed for permission to reprint excerpts from the following previously published material:

Contents

CONTENTS

SHAME AND THE SELF

·I·

Introduction

• 1 •

Overview

The fall in the Genesis myth of Adam and Eve was accompanied by the introduction of shame into the experience of mankind. Prior to the eating of the forbidden fruit "they were both naked and they were not ashamed." It was the acquisition of a *special kind of knowledge*, designated in Genesis as the knowledge of good and evil, that was the occasion of the fall and the first appearance of shame. With the eating of the fruit and the acquisition of that special kind of knowing

> Then the eyes of both of them were opened, and they knew they were naked; and they sewed fig leaves together and made themselves coverings.
>
> And they heard the sound of the Lord God walking in the garden in the cool of the day, and Adam and his wife hid themselves from the presence of the Lord God among the trees of the garden.
>
> Then the Lord God called to Adam and said to him "Where are you?"
>
> So he said "I heard Your voice in the garden and I was afraid because I was naked; and I hid myself."
>
> And He said "Who told you that you were naked? Have you eaten from the tree of which I commanded you that you should not eat? (Genesis 3:7–11, King James Translation)

Adam's confessed awareness of his nakedness is for God incontrovertible evidence of the acquisition of objective self-awareness. With the acquisition of objective self-awareness comes shame and the need for concealment. The exploration of

3

this connection between objective self-awareness and shame will occupy us in the pages to follow.

Smith (1984) quotes Schuon (1965) on Adam's fall: "The link with the divine Source was broken and became invisible, the world became suddenly external to Adam, things became opaque and heavy, they became like unintelligible and hostile fragments" (p. 44). And Smith adds, "In other words, the world *as we know it* came into existence: history began" (p. 156, emphasis added). The Genesis myth thus suggests that history began with shame and the suddenly altered perception of the world associated with that shame. As something now external, opaque, and heavy, the world had to be probed, seen through, and weighed; as unintelligible, it had to be studied and researched; as hostile, it had to be subdued, controlled, or destroyed. We recognize this as the worldview of empirical science. It is not my intention in this book to critique modern science, however, but rather to present a theory of shame embedded in a better understanding of the nature of self experience.

Shame is an experience that has not been much talked about in contemporary society, although that situation is currently changing. One might almost say that there has been a cultural conspiracy to avoid discussing shame. When friends and acquaintances learned that I was writing a book, they would invariably ask about the subject of the book; when I replied that I was writing about shame, a frequent response was "Oh," followed either by an awkward silence or a prompt change of subject. Shame, as Lewis (1987) noted, makes us want to hide; we avert our gaze and hang our head in shame. Shame is so painful that we hope it ends quickly; we have no particular desire to reflect on it or talk about it, because to do so is to run the risk of reexperiencing it. Shame is also somewhat contagious; it is difficult to witness another person's acute shame or embarrassment without some vicarious twinge in ourselves. Exploring others' feelings of shame puts us in touch with our own unacknowledged or unmastered shame. We tend to be ashamed of being ashamed and try to deny and hide our shame for that reason.

In the past decade a number of important articles and books on shame have appeared, testifying to an increasing awareness of the importance of shame as a pathogenic force in the develop-

4

ment and maintenance of various clinical disorders. Shame and defenses against shame have been implicated as playing crucial roles in such varied conditions as depression, manic–depressive illness, schizophrenia, eating disorders, personality disorders, social phobias (Bursten, 1973; Lewis, 1987; Morrison, 1989; Wurmser, 1981), addictions (Fossum & Mason, 1986), and sexual perversions (Stoller, 1987). Shame is also intimately involved in complex affective states such as rage, envy, despair, hopelessness, contempt (Morrison, 1989; Wurmser 1981), vanity, conceit, ambition, pride, and ruthlessness (Broucek, 1982; Nathanson, 1987a).

I believe it was the eminent physician William Osler who said that if one really knew syphilis one knew medicine. This was, of course, in the pre-antibiotic days when unsuccessfully treated syphilis could present in a variety of ways, affecting many organ systems and requiring of the physician extensive knowledge of differential diagnosis. In my own clinical work I have come to the conclusion that if one knows shame one knows psychopathology (and also something about health).

Throughout this book the word shame will be used in four different ways: (1) as it is used in common everyday parlance; (2) to designate an innate affect; (3) to designate a category or family of "feelings," all assumed to be variants of the same underlying innate affect (these experiences include what we refer to in our everyday language of emotion as shyness, reticence, embarrassment, chagrin, painful self-consciousness, feelings of inferiority and inadequacy, mortification, disgrace, and dishonor); and (4) to refer to "the sense of shame" or anticipatory shame, that is, the discretionary function that makes us pause before saying or doing something that would arouse the painful feeling of shame in ourselves or another. This distinction between the sense of shame and an actual shame experience is not made by most writers on shame. Carl Schneider (1977) has drawn needed attention to this neglected distinction and has emphasized how vital is the sense of shame to our individual and collective emotional, moral, and spiritual welfare. The clinical literature on shame is focused on shame as affect and usually fails to recognize the concept of the sense of shame as the safeguard of our psychic life.

5

There seem to be so many potential sources of shame that it is difficult to identify common denominators. One may be ashamed of almost anything about oneself—one's appearance, dress, mannerisms, bodily characteristics, personality traits, and so forth. One may be ashamed at times of anything with which one feels in any way identified—one's ethnic origins, country, religion, family, etc. One may feel shame over failure to be accepted or valued by any person or group whose acceptance is desired. Any perceived loss of love or respect from a loved one may trigger shame. One may feel shame over a lack of competence or over the loss of previously acquired competence, as might occur with illness or aging. Any loss of control over one's body, mental functions, or emotions may elicit shame. In childhood any loss of sphincter control after continence has been achieved is apt to be accompanied by shame, regardless of whether there is any overt shaming response from others. Shame often has to do with matters of exposure when one is not prepared for such exposure. When personal boundaries are not respected by others, shame and shame rage are apt to be the result. Shame also has to do with one's relationship to one's bodily functions and may be elicited under certain circumstances in association with eating, excretion, and sexuality. Anytime the self experiences itself as ruled by some "lower" passion, the self may be vulnerable to shame. Failure to measure up to what others expect or what one expects of oneself may elicit shame.

Although this brief inventory of possible occasions for shame is by no means exhaustive, it does perhaps give some sense of the range of sources involved. The shame arising from the aforementioned sources is not always consciously felt and properly identified by the person who is experiencing the affect of shame. The affect of shame may be activated without the feeling of shame. Basch (1983, 1988) distinguishes between affect, feeling, and emotion. He reserves the term *affect* for those innate, involuntary somatic reactions that provide the physiological underpinning for feeling and emotion. Basch (1988) drew for his understanding of affect on the work of Tomkins (1962, 1963), who identified nine innate affects (see Chapter 2). Affects are, in a sense, "prepsychological" and can be observed in the neonate. *Feeling* is the developmentally more advanced (18–

6

24 months) conscious awareness of an affective event as a subjective experience belonging to the self. *Emotion*, in Basch's view,
refers to more complex states involving the joining of feeling
states with personal experience to give rise to states such as love,
hate, and happiness. Although I do not fully subscribe to these
distinctions that Basch makes, he is right in pointing out that
affects may or may not be consciously registered as "feelings"
even when the capacity for such awareness is present. More
frequently than not, shame affect is unrecognized and unarticulated. We can differentiate three different types of shame experience (Lewis 1971, 1987): (1) overt, consciously experienced
and acknowledged shame, characteristically accompanied by a
lowering of the head, averted gaze, blushing, an acute sense of
confusion, and painful self-consciousness; (2) overt unidentified
or unacknowledged shame, in which case the person shows
unmistakable signs of a shame reaction but does not consciously
recognize or acknowledge the shame affect he or she is experiencing; and (3) bypassed shame, in which case the person is obviously dealing with a shaming event and may refer to feeling
embarrassed, but without strong shame feeling, except for a brief
jolt to the self—and deals with the shame experience by incessant, obsessive ideation about the role of the self in the shaming
event.

Because shame seems so intimately connected with the self,
a better understanding of shame would seem to promise a better
understanding of the self. Shame suggests that the self is a
relational and contextual structure; it is dependent on the maintenance of coordinates (in the form of networks of relationships
and identifications, conscious and unconscious, early and recent) locating us firmly in the interpersonal field. The concept of
the atomistic isolated self is a delusion that assumes because the
body is a discrete mass of limited extension that the self and
psyche are also. Consider the term *intrapsychic*; implicit in this
term is the metaphor of psyche as container. Writers who use the
term often seem unaware of the metaphorical nature of this
notion and consider the psyche to have literal boundaries that
are tacitly or explicitly regarded as equivalent to the boundaries
of the brain.

Much has been made by some theorists of the distinction

between the intrapsychic and the interpersonal as it relates to shame and guilt. According to these theorists, the capacity to experience guilt represents a higher level of superego development than does the experience of shame. Singer (Piers & Singer, 1953) settled this issue to my satisfaction when he marked off the following parallel levels of shame and guilt:

> (a) Feelings of shame or guilt aroused in the physical presence of an audience; (b) feelings of shame or guilt aroused in the mental presence of an audience, i.e., in the presence of a phantasy or "eidetic" audience; (c) feelings of shame or guilt aroused without conscious or "realistic" reference to an actual or imaginary audience and presumably representing a reactivation of anxieties originally aroused in childhood by parental disapproval or punishment; and (d) feelings of shame and guilt aroused without conscious reference to a physical or a phantasy audience and presumably depending only on abstract moral principles accepted by the self. (p. 76)

Of Singer's parallel levels of shame and guilt, (a) would be considered by many theorists to lie in the interpersonal realm and (b), (c), and (d) would be presumably intrapsychic, but I find it more useful to think of these levels in terms of the concretely interpersonal, the memorialized interpersonal, and the abstractly interpersonal; that way we avoid the spurious dichotomy between the intrapsychic and the interpersonal. But even if one insists on the usefulness of the terms *intrapsychic* and *internalized*, it is still the case that both shame and guilt may be more or less internalized and thus more or less intrapsychic.

A few remarks about the plan of this book. After presenting a critical review of the theoretical and clinical literature on shame in Part I, I present in Part II a theory of shame embedded in a larger theory of the development of the self. I attempt to show that shame is closely tied to the developing sense of self and reflects a disturbance in the interpersonal matrix out of which that sense of self develops. A major focus in this first section will be on shame as a response to objectification, that is, as a response to having one's status as a subject ignored, disregarded, denied, or negated. Such objectifications sever what Kaufman (1985) has called "the interpersonal bridge."

In Part III, dealing with interpersonal dimensions of shame, we look at the ways in which individuals and groups inflict shame on certain persons and the reasons why they do so. We then examine the way in which psychoanalysis and much psychotherapy, by virtue of the way they are set up and conducted, tend to evoke, enhance, and augment shame (for both parties) while the practitioner remains insufficiently aware of the shame-inducing conditions operating in his or her consulting room.

Part IV expands the focus of our study to include an analysis of the impact on our society of the dissemination of psychoanalytic views and attitudes concerning shame. The relationship between shame and sexuality is reexamined and radically revised. The problem of modern shamelessness is then explored and this exploration includes an excursion into the evolution of modern consciousness as that consciousness has been shaped by the invention of the camera and all its modern descendants.

We begin our study by surveying the efforts of various theorists and investigators to understand shame, starting with Freud. The following review is admittedly selective, highlighting certain contributions and undoubtedly neglecting others.

·2·

A Critical Review
of the Literature on Shame

EARLY PSYCHOANALYTIC CONTRIBUTIONS
TO AN UNDERSTANDING OF SHAME

To get our bearings in this field we might first consider Freud's ideas about shame. In his "Three Essays on the Theory of Sexuality," Freud (1905/1953) spoke of shame and disgust as barriers to the instinctual life, barriers that have been exploited in the service of the child's cultural and moral education by those entrusted with that responsibility. Although Freud believed shame to be "organically determined and fixed by heredity" (p. 177), his fondness for Lamarckian notions about the inheritance of acquired characteristics and his vision of natural man led him to speculate that in the early history of the race man was unashamed and that shame came about as the precipitate of external inhibitions against instinctual gratification. In the historical sequence of what Freud calls "the psychogenesis of the human race" (p. 162), the unbridled expression of instinctual drives was followed by acquired inhibition, which eventually modified the germ plasm and became genetically transmitted as the now innate affect of shame. According to Freud, both phylogenetically and ontogenetically, shame is reactive, inhibitory, and prohibitive, opposing the pleasure principle and leading one to abstain from certain (more natural) behaviors; man's primary condition is shameless or unashamed. Shame and disgust are

11

seen as promoting repression, but they do not thereby alter the character or persistence of the original drive component being repressed.

In the "Three Essays on the Theory of Sexuality," Freud introduces the idea that in the development of the child shame is most closely allied with the "partial drive" or "component instinct" of scopophilia, the love of looking—more specifically, sexually oriented looking. Why such a connection? Freud does not venture an explanation.

In his 1930 essay on "Civilization and its Discontents" Freud suggests that shame originated when man, in his evolution, first acquired the upright posture: "this made his genitals, which were previously concealed, visible and in need of protection, and so provoked feelings of shame in him" (p. 99). This idea clearly conflicts with his earlier view of shame as the precipitate of external inhibitions against instinctual gratification. In his "New Introductory Lectures on Psychoanalysis" Freud (1933/1964) goes on to relate shame not so much to a need to hide and protect the genitals but to conceal genital deficiency. Shame thus became "a feminine characteristic *par excellence*" (p. 132).

In summary, Freud had no consistent theory of shame. Shame received relatively little attention in the Freudian corpus, especially as contrasted with anxiety or guilt. I attempt to show in later chapters that Freud's attitude and the attitude of later psychoanalysts toward shame was one of disrespect. Shame was viewed as one of the major forces promoting repression and resistance to the analytic process, thus opposing insight into the sexual dynamics underlying the various neuroses.

Psychoanalysts Fenichel (1945) and Nunberg (1955), echoing Freud's ideas about the link between shame and the scopophilic drive, emphasized the relationship between exhibitionism (the passive form of scopophilia, according to Freud) and shame, viewing shame as a reaction formation to exhibitionistic wishes. As Spiegal (1966) noted, however, "The usual derivation of shame from the repression of exhibitionistic drives does not coincide with the observation that shame can appear before such repression has taken place" (p. 86). Miller (1985) says of the theorists who view shame as a reaction formation against exhibitionism: "Although they identify the commonplace situation in which shame experience interrupts morally forbidden exhibitionism, they mistake that function for the defining core of the shame experience. One can prop open a window with a book but that does not mean a book is essentially a window prop" (p. 11).

LATER PSYCHOANALYTIC CONTRIBUTIONS TO AN UNDERSTANDING OF SHAME

Any survey of psychoanalytic theories of shame must include Erikson's (1950) work on identity and the life cycle, in which he linked shame to anal phase struggles involving self-control and autonomy. Whether shame and self-doubt become more or less permanent features of the personality depends, according to Erikson, on the interpersonal dynamics surrounding anal phase issues and the extent to which the child's sense of autonomy is damaged during that phase of development. Erikson outlined eight stages in the life cycle, which he designated by contrasting negative and positive emotional outcomes; they were, in developmental sequence, basic trust versus basic mistrust, autonomy versus shame and doubt, initiative versus guilt, industry versus inferiority, identity versus role confusion, intimacy versus isolation, generativity versus stagnation, ego integrity versus despair. Kaufman (1989) astutely noted that "the negative pole of each crisis is actually an elaboration of shame, given new or wider meaning. Each subsequent crisis involves, at least in part, a reworking of shame" (p. 10).

Another important psychoanalytic contributor to our understanding of shame was Piers (Piers & Singer, 1953), who conceptualized shame as reflecting a tension between ego and ego-ideal due to a discrepancy between the actual state of the ego and the ego-ideal. Piers carefully distinguished between guilt and shame. He saw guilt as having to do with transgression and shame with failure. According to Piers, the unconscious threat implied in shame was abandonment, in guilt castration. Piers also described shame-guilt cycles (which are of great clinical importance) and made important observations about shame-guilt dynamics in masochism.

Levin (1967), in an important essay on shame, suggested

13

that shame was "a basic component of the normal homeostatic mechanisms regulating the sexual drive" (p. 270). He proposed that the function of shame was to direct the sexual drive away from danger and protect one from the trauma of overexposure to others with its attendant risk of rejection. From the perspective of the present study, what Levin described was the function of *the sense of shame*, or protective shame, rather than the function of the affect shame. Ideas similar to Levin's concerning the role of shame in the normal regulation of the sexual drive were earlier put forward by the philosopher Max Scheler (1913), and we examine those ideas in a later chapter.

Levin also introduced the distinction between primary and secondary shame: secondary shame is shame about shame. As Levin points out, an individual who manifests little evidence of shame is often admired for his "strength." People tend to hide their shame from others and from themselves because they are ashamed of their vulnerability to shame affect. Thus we see "countershame" character traits in many people, such as the stereotypical "macho" male.

RECENT PSYCHOANALYTIC CONTRIBUTIONS

Wurmser (1981), while making many sensitive and important observations about shame, continued in the classical psychoanalytic tradition of deriving shame from conflicts involving the *partial drives* of voyeurism and exhibitionism. He proposed more archaic and more general forms of these drives, which he labeled "theatophilia" (corresponding to voyeurism) and "delophilia" (exhibitionism). Theatophilia was defined as the desire to watch and observe, to be fascinated, and to merge and master through attentive looking. Delophilia was defined as the drive for self-expression and the desire to fascinate others by one's self exposure—that is, to show and impress, to merge with the other through communication.

According to Wurmser, the theatophilic drive originates in the "zone" of the perceptual organs, especially the eye, and its aim is merger with its object, which is a powerful gripping "configuration" or person. Its mode is curious attention; its

14

accompanying affects are admiration and awe and, if successfully consummated, enthusiasm and joy. If the drive is blocked in its gratification, shame anxiety results—the fear of being "petrified" by the look of the object. Delophilia, the expressive, exhibitionistic drive, originates in the "zone" of expressive organs (the face, especially eyes and mouth); its aim is to fascinate and overpower the other person or persons. Its accompanying affect is pride, and if the drive is successful, a sense of glory, grandeur, and ecstatic self-confidence ensues. Its mode is expressive communication. If the drive is thwarted, the negative affects of contempt for the other and/or shame (as self-contempt) ensue.

By means of these formulations Wurmser attempted to conserve and extend the basic Freudian understanding of shame as derivative of conflict involving exhibitionistic and voyeuristic partial drives, and also conserve the Freudian notion that component drives are linked to libidinal zones. By so doing Wurmser tried to show that the theoretical views of psychoanalyst Heinz Kohut and his school of "self psychology" could be more adequately formulated within the framework of classical Freudian drive theory, as extended and elaborated by Wurmser.

Although I will not attempt to discuss Kohut's theoretical formulations in any depth in this introductory survey chapter, I will briefly sketch some of his ideas for the reader who may not be familiar with his work in order to promote an understanding of Wurmser's critique of Kohutian theory. Kohut (1971) postulated a bipolar self consisting of the grandiose self as one pole and the idealized "selfobject" as the other. The grandiose self requires adequate mirroring on the part of the significant caregiving and nurturing figures in the course of the child's early development if that development is to proceed optimally. Lacking adequate mirroring, the child has a second chance to establish a strong and cohesive self if one of the significant caregiving others will lend himself or herself to serve as an idealized selfobject. The selfobject, as the name implies, is experienced as both other and as part of the self.

Wurmser views the grandiose self as coordinated with the delophilic drive, and the idealized selfobject with the theatophilic drive. Delophilia involves the desire to overwhelm the

15

other by the magical power of one's expression, that is, the desire to charm, fascinate, mesmerize. In theatophilia, one is enthralled with the awe-inspiring other and submits to the magic power of the other to charm and enrich. In Wurmser's view, Kohut's bipolar self can be better understood in terms of these two "drives."

Despite Wurmser's unhappiness with Kohut's formulations he and Kohut both linked shame to drive theory and thus stayed within the classical psychoanalytic view of shame as a derivative of the scopophilic instinct. Kohut maintained that shame is the result of the flooding of the ego with "unneutralized" exhibition-ism and thus represents an "economic" disturbance in libidinal discharge.

Morrison (1989) has taken issue with Kohut's narrow view of the nature of shame in narcissistic disorders and has instead opted for a modified version of Piers's (1953) idea that shame is reflective of tension between the ego and the ego-ideal. Morrison translates Piers's structural terms into the language of self psy-chology, resulting in the restatement that shame reflects severe tension or strain between the self and the ideal self. We take a closer look at Morrison's work when we discuss shame and narcissism in a later chapter.

Lewis (1988), drawing on the attachment theory of Bowlby and others and on neurophysiological investigations of the sepa-ration–distress system, emphasizes a relationship between shame and separation distress/panic. According to Lewis, "Vicarious emotional experience is the foundation of attachment on both sides. . . . Shame is the empathic or vicarious experience of the other's rejection of the self. Shame is the state in which one accepts the loss of the other as if it were a loss in the self" (p. 103).

Another contribution of Lewis (1971), mentioned in Chap-ter 1, is the distinction she draws, based on psychotherapy material, between (1) overt acknowledged shame, (2) overt un-identified or unacknowledged shame, such as in the case of a person who is in an acute state of self-hatred but does not recognize or acknowledge the affect of shame; and (3) bypassed shame. In the case of bypassed shame, the person is clearly dealing with shaming events but is not caught up in shame

16

feeling, except for a momentary jolt to the self; instead, the person seems to be dealing with shame experiences by incessant ideation about the role of the self in the shaming events.

IS SHAME A SPECIAL PROBLEM
FOR PSYCHOANALYSIS?

How are we to understand the relative neglect of shame in earlier psychoanalytic literature and the failure of psychoanalysis until relatively recently to attempt to develop a consistent theory of shame? Aside from the fact that psychoanalysis has lacked a satisfactory general theory of affect, I think there are many other reasons for the state of affairs as regards shame. Some of these reasons will be explored in a later chapter on shame, psychoanalysis and psychotherapy (Chapter 7). Here I will mention only two—the first having to do with Freud's personality and his own unanalyzed shame issues, the second having to do with the early history of the psychoanalytic movement.

Roustang (1986) contrasts psychoanalytic theory with what he calls "genuinely scientific theories" and notes that a biologist could understand the theory of Watson and Crick without knowing anything about them as persons but a psychoanalyst needs to take Freud's personality into account if he is to understand anything of psychoanalytic theory. As Rousting says, "the study of psychoanalysis cannot be separated from the peculiarities of Freud's psyche" (p. 60). Several writers (Mannoni, 1982; Morrison, 1989; Tomkins, 1963) have highlighted shame issues as being of particular importance in Freud's early development and personality structure and it would appear that his self-analysis bypassed these shame issues in favor of an emphasis on guilt.

When I say that a second reason for the absence of an adequate theory of shame had to do with the early history of the psychoanalytic movement, I am referring to the group dynamics governing the relationship between Freud and his circle of disciples. More specifically, I am referring to the question of how much deviation from the Master's line of thought was permissible if one was to remain a member of that inner circle. As

Roustang (1986) notes, a comparison of Freud's analysis of the Church and the Army in "Group Psychology and the Analysis of the Ego" (1921/1955) with his project for a psychoanalytic society in "On the History of the Psycho-analytic Movement" (1914/1957) reveals very similar themes: loyalty and devotion to the founder, allegiance to the leader, faithful adherence to one doctrine, rejection of dissidents, and so forth. The losses that Freud's circle of disciples ("the savage hoard," as Freud called them) incurred as the result of the the expulsion of dissidents is all too well known to require extensive review here.

Groups use both guilt and shame to ensure conformity to group norms. Piers (1953) makes the point that social conformity achieved through guilt will be a conformity based on submission, with punishment as the threat. Social conformity achieved through shame will be essentially a conformity based on identification and shared ideals, with rejection, expulsion, or abandonment as the threat. It seems clear that the conformity achieved within Freud's circle of disciples was primarily of the latter type. Shame anxiety underlies the conformity within such a group. Because the cohesiveness of the psychoanalytic movement was based on shame anxiety, it is not surprising that guilt received so much attention from Freud (and subsequent generations of analysts) and shame so little. The function of shame and shame anxiety in maintaining the group identification with Freud had to remain unanalyzed if Freud was to fashion and maintain the type of group he envisioned. On the eve of their final break Adler complained of "the nonsensical castration" that Freud intended to perform publicly on him "before everyone's eyes" (Gay, 1988). *Castration* is here obviously a code word for humiliation, as is often the case in the psychoanalytic literature.

Adler's emphasis on inferiority feelings and "masculine protest" pointed toward the importance of shame. Morrison (1989) wrote, "One need not fully endorse Adler's formulations to see how close they come to a framework that would allow for shame and its manifestations (although, interestingly, Adler himself never did so)" (p. 4). Morrison suggests that Freud's conflict with Adler may have been another factor that contributed to his subsequent neglect of shame.

CONTRIBUTIONS TO AN UNDERSTANDING OF SHAME FROM OUTSIDE PSYCHOANALYSIS

Lynd

Lynd's (1958) book *On Shame and the Search for Identity* presented a remarkably lucid exposition of the nature of the shame experience. She teased out the following aspects of that experience:

1. Exposure, particularly unexpected exposure, to others usually but even more importantly to ourselves. Blushing is a manifestation of the involuntary, unexpected nature of the shame experience, which makes one want to cover the face, hide, disappear. A sense of confusion accompanies this sudden unexpected exposure.

2. Incongruity or inappropriateness. "In shame experience what is exposed is incongruous with or glaringly inappropriate to the situation or it violates our previous image of ourselves" (p. 34). This suddenly experienced incongruity may have to do with relatively inconsequential matters.

> It is the very triviality of the cause—an awkward gesture, a gaucherie in dress or table manners, "an untimely joke" always "a source of bitter regret," a gift or a witticism that falls flat, an expressed naivete in taste, a mispronounced word, ignorance of some unimportant detail that everyone else knows—that helps to give shame its unbearable character. (p. 40)

3. Threat to trust. In shame experience trust is seriously jeopardized or sometimes destroyed. This may result in doubts about one's adequacy or in questioning the values of the immediate world around oneself. "Sudden experience of a violation of expectation, of incongruity between expectation and outcome, results in a shattering of trust in oneself, even in one's own body and skill and identity, and in the trusted boundaries or framework of the society and the world one has known" (p. 46). The

meaningfulness of life and the world order may be thrown into doubt and a heightened sense of tragedy may result.

4. Involvement of the whole self. Guilt involves a "culturally defined wrong act, a part of oneself that is separable, segmented and redeemable. But an experience of shame . . . cannot be modified by addition, or wiped out by subtraction, or exorcised by expiation. It is not an isolated act that can be detached from the self" (p. 50). Shame involves one's core sense of identity.

5. Difficulty in communicating shame. All of the previously listed characteristics of experiences of shame make such experiences almost impossible to communicate.

Tomkins

The affect theorist Silvan Tomkins (1963) devoted considerable attention to shame in his magnum opus *Affect, Imagery, and Consciousness, Vol. II* and more recently (1987) in his contribution to *The Many Faces of Shame*, edited by Donald Nathanson. The radically different feature of Tomkins's approach to shame is that it is not based on drive theory but on a fully developed theory of affects, which is still insufficiently known and appreciated. Tomkins's theory of shame was employed and elaborated upon by Nathanson (1987b) in his own contribution to the same volume, in which he attempted to outline a developmental timetable for shame. Kaufman (1985, 1989; see next section of this chapter) also draws on Tomkins's theory of shame. Any effort to develop a more unified theory of shame must take into account Tomkins' ideas about shame.

Tomkins has identified nine discrete innate affects, which he sees as controlled by inherited subcortical "programs" that, in turn, control facial muscle responses, autonomic blood flow, and respiratory and vocal responses. These innate affects include (1) two positive affects: interest–excitement and enjoyment–joy; (2) six negative affects: fear, anger, distress, shame, dismell (affective reaction to noxious odors), and disgust; and (3) one resetting affect, surprise. Except for dismell and disgust, which Tomkins sees as drive auxiliaries (i.e., regulating the oral drive by guarding against the ingestion of noxious substances), and shame which Tomkins labels an "affect auxillary" the other affects are activated by various profiles of "neural firing."

According to Tomkins (1963, 1987), the innate activator of shame is an incomplete reduction of interest–excitement or enjoyment–joy. Since Shame, in Tomkins's view, is an affect auxillary (that is to say, it is not a basic affect, per se, but is auxillary to the affects of interest–excitement and enjoyment–joy), any barrier to the ongoing experience of interest-excitement or enjoyment-joy that dampens but does not destroy such interest or enjoyment may activate shame. Although Tomkins's formula seems to fit very nicely with a great many shame experiences, it has the weakness that one can, without too much difficulty, think of numerous instances in which the formula apparently fails to hold. For example, one is watching, with great interest and excitement, a sporting event on TV when a technical problem briefly interrupts the transmission of the picture. One may feel distressed or enraged about this turn of events—but ashamed? Neither introspection nor observation of others confirms that shame is ordinarily activated in such a situation but, according to Tomkins's formula, it ought to be. Or imagine oneself enjoying a delicious meal when one's dinner companion shares some disconcerting information that dampens one's enjoyment of the meal. Is one likely to experience shame in such a situation? I think not.

It seems indisputable that shame is about the self and its social context and is reflective of a disturbance in the sense of self as well as a disturbance in the nature of the relationship with the other. In Tomkins's writings one finds curious contradictions on this issue. In his most recent writing on shame, Tomkins (1987) maintains that "shame is in no way limited to the self, to the other, or to society" (p. 153). In his earlier (1963) work on shame Tomkins wrote, "In contrast to all other affects, shame is an experience of the self by the self. At that moment when the self feels ashamed, it is felt as a sickness within the self. Shame is the most reflexive of affects in that the phenomenological distinction between the subject and object of shame is lost" (p. 133). Running through much of Tomkins earlier writing on shame is an emphasis on shame as resulting from an impediment to interpersonal communication. I believe this to be one of the most important contributions that Tomkins has made to our understanding of shame, along with the idea that in the shame response the self remains positively committed to the other or to that part of the self that has created an impediment to communication. Shame implies the wish to maintain or restore the "good" relationship. We shall consider Tomkins's ideas about shame again in the next chapter when we explore the development of the sense of self in infancy and try to determine when the affect of shame makes its first appearance in the developing child.

Other Contributions to an Understanding of Shame

Kaufman (1985, 1989), who has written extensively on shame, draws on Tomkins's shame theory. While accepting the idea that shame is activated by the incomplete reduction of interest or enjoyment, Kaufman emphasizes an "interpersonal activator," which is a rupture of the "interpersonal bridge," an emotional bond established between individuals based on shared positive affect, communicative understanding, mutual valuing, and respect. When one individual somehow breaks the interpersonal bridge with the other, shame is generated. In positing an interpersonal activator, Kaufman is drawing on Tomkins's earlier emphasis on shame as resulting from an impediment to communication with a positively valued other.

If shame is a response to rejection or the breaking of the interpersonal bridge, it is not clear precisely why these events should result in the painful feeling of exposure with the concomitant wish to hide. This is an example of a recurrent problem in existing theories of shame; no theory about the causes, sources, or mechanisms of shame adequately accounts for all characteristics of the shame experience. Relating shame to scopophilic drives fails to explain the relationship of shame to self, ideals, and identity (as Thrane, 1979, points out) or why it is so central to self-esteem regulation. The same could be said about the notion that shame is activated by a partial reduction of the affects of interest and excitement.

Nathanson (1987b), drawing on Tomkins's affect theory

and specifically on Tomkins's ideas about shame as resulting from the existence of an obstacle to interest–excitement or enjoyment–joy that dampens or attenuates those affects, attempts to account for the close relationship between shame and the self and shame and sexuality as, essentially, developmentally *learned* relationships, as Tomkins's theory would require. My basic assumption is that shame is *innately* connected to the sense of self and to sexuality, as put forth in subsequent chapters.

Nathanson also links shame and interest–excitement to manic–depressive illness and presents a novel and intriguing theory of manic–depressive illness as involving a neurophysiological dysregulation of the affects of interest–excitement and shame.

For Schneider (1977) the core of the shame experience is found in the sense of visibility and exposure. One of Schneider's most important insights is his recognition that it is a *special kind of visibility* and exposure that is at the core of shame experience. Schneider notes that the word *expose* is derived from the Latin *exponere*, which means "to put out" or "to place out," suggesting a spatial context in which things have their proper place and proper fit. Schneider says, "we experience shame when we feel we are placed out of the context within which we wish to be interpreted" (p. 35). This insight will be pivotal in much of what follows. We examine the nature of this special kind of visibility and exposure in Chapters 3 and 4. Schneider, as mentioned in the previous chapter, has also drawn much needed attention to the fact that a well-developed sense of shame protects us from gratuitous over-exposure at the times when we are most vulnerable.

Straus (1980), like Schneider, also makes much of the important protective function of the sense of shame—particularly for the adolescent for whom the delicate and necessarily private unfinished process of psychosexual maturation is in need of protection from premature public exposure in the adult world of the already completed. Thus shame is a safeguard against violation of incest prohibitions. "Shame is a protection against the public in all of its forms," says Straus (p. 222).

Straus also rejects the Freudian notion of partial drives or component sexual drives, at least as far as voyeurism and exhibitionism are concerned. He maintains that voyeurism (and, by implication, exhibitionism also) is not a "normal" component of the sexual drive but instead reflects an alteration in communicative mode, involving distancing and objectification (more about that in Chapter 9, which is devoted to a reassessment of the relationship between shame and sexuality and in Chapter 10, devoted to understanding modern shamelessness).

SOME CONCLUDING REMARKS

This admittedly incomplete survey of the modern literature on shame should at least convey to the reader some of the areas of agreement and disagreement about the affect of shame, its functions, and its relationship to sexuality, self, and other. It should also be apparent that there is considerable controversy about the basic nature of shame and the role shame plays in our psychic life.

The next three chapters are grouped together under the part heading *Shame and the Formation of the Self*. First I present some theoretical ideas about the sense of self. I propose that the earliest source of shame is the infant's experiences of inefficacy, particularly interpersonal inefficacy, the experience of failure to competently initiate and sustain mutually gratifying inter-subjectivity or shared consciousness. The second source of shame, developmentally speaking, is self-objectification, a process that brings about a kind of self-alienation or primary disso-ciation (described in Chapter 4). A third source of shame is the episodic or chronic experience of being unloved, rejected, or scapegoated by important others (parents, primarily). In the course of development these sources of shame bring about the self's overinvestment in the idealized self-image and a devalu-ation of the actual self, a development that is the focus of Chapter 5 "Shame and Narcississm."

·II·

Shame and the Formation of the Self

·3·

The Sense of Self

Disturbances in the sense of self underlie various psychopatho-logical conditions. One of the obstacles to a coherent theory of self has been the failure to adequately conceptualize what it is that we refer to when we talk about self-feeling or the sense of self, terms I shall be using as synonyms in what follows. In earlier work (1977, 1979, 1982) I developed the thesis that the earliest sense of self grows out of the experience of efficacy, fulfilled intentionality, and the joy and excitement attendant on that experience. The sense of self at the bodily level is grounded in patterns of kinesthetic "flows" that flesh out volitional activity. As Zaner (1981) observes, the feeling of these kinesthetic "flows" is

> what *most fundamentally consitutes this body as my embodiment.* They continuously function in a *double manner*: on the one hand, they enact, concretely "flesh-out," the rudimentary strivings, efforts, wishings, and wantings; on the other, what-ever appears in any of the sensory fields is strictly, *functionally correlated* to the actualizing of these kinaesthetic flow-patterns. These, too, reveal an *"if/then"* pattern: "if" I move my arm in specific ways, "then" the glass is knocked off the table. Thus *bodily experience at its roots, and not only in relation to resistant or impacting objects, has this "causal" style* . . . kinaesthetic flows are the *"urgefuhlt'"* of bodily life, at once embodying mental strivings and positioning or orienting the appearing of other objects . . . They are *essentially "means"*; kinaesthetic patterns are that by virtue of which anything else is able to appear or be experienced. (pp. 42–43)

Jonas (1966) points out that the experiential source of the concept of causality "is not regular connection, not even necessary connection, but force and influence; . . . the source of this experience is, indeed, not sense perception, but our body exerting itself in action "(p. 33). The source of the concept of energy is also rooted in the same experience. Our scientific understanding of the physical world in terms of force, causality, energy, and space has its roots in this experience of our bodily strivings. The application of these concepts to the physical world involves metaphorical projections of schemata emerging from bodily experience (see Johnson, 1987, for a further exposition of this subject).

The "causal" style of bodily experience contributes significantly to the infant's development of a sense of self based on efficacy or "agency." Thus, a rudimentary sense of self is present from the earliest days of life. It is manifested very early in what Tomkins (1981) has called "autosimulation," the infant's voluntary imitation of his/her own reflexes. Not long after birth the infant will replace reflex sucking with voluntary sucking and reflex visual tracking with voluntary tracking. Tomkins insists that from the first moments of life infants are engaged in making good scenes better by *doing it themselves*. Autosimulation is one of the first manifestations of intent, and this intent is supported from the first by the innate affects of interest–excitement and enjoyment. Intent, as I use the term, has to do with knowing what one is doing and why and involves, even in the infant, a degree of what might be called "willing." As Jonas (1974) points out, every willing wills itself, and thus there is an inherent reflexiveness in the operations of the will. Out of this intentionality and its inherent reflexiveness, its success or efficacy, and the positive affects attendant on that success, the sense of self will form. The kinesthetic flows that constitute the bodily foundation for this intentionality are the core experiences out of which the sense of self at the physical level emerges.

The efficacy of the infant's efforts vis-à-vis the world obviously depends on sensitive and "good enough" maternal responsiveness. To the extent that the mother–child interaction fails to support and sustain a sense of efficacy, the primitive sense of self will be damaged, and the capacity for initiative may

28

be nipped in the bud, leading to a more or less robotic type of existence in which the child, as he grows older, attempts to establish a compensatory sense of self by the suppression or repression of his original action tendencies, based on an identification with the mother ("mother" is to be understood as shorthand for the primary caretaker or caretakers). In other words, the sense of self, if not based on effective interaction and communication with other persons, may instead become based on effective inhibitory activities in relation to oneself. Thus, with certain patients one cannot modify their defenses without also seriously disturbing their sense of self and producing profound depersonalization experiences.

In an earlier paper (1979), I reviewed a number of experimental studies, the "contingency" studies, that dealt with the infant's control (or lack of control) over environmental events, studies that clearly demonstrated the infant's excitement, and near insatiability in recreating events contingent on his/her activity. For example, the 4-month-old infants in the "switching on" experiments of Papousek and Papousek (1975) had to find out by themselves and by chance that rotating the head at least 30 degrees to a predetermined side would activate a multicolored light display. Before the experiments the light display was attractive to the infants, but after several repetitions habituation would occur and they would show less interest in the display. When the light display was contingent on the infants' activities and the infants grasped that fact, their behavior changed dramatically. They insatiably repeated the behavior "with such joyful affect in . . . gestures and vocalization that it seemed more like attachment than habituation" (p. 252). The infants in these studies also exhibited a negative affect state associated with the inability to influence, predict, or comprehend an event that they expected, on the basis of previous experience, to be able to control or understand. The description of the behavioral and physiological characteristics of these negative affect states led me to consider these states as primitive shame experiences.

On the basis of these studies and other observations, I posited that efficacy experience or fulfilled intent, driven by the innate affect of interest–excitement (see discussion of Tomkins's

29

affect theory in Chapter 2) and rewarded by enjoyment–joy, was the basis for the formation of a healthy sense of self and healthy "pride" (see Nathanson, 1987a, on the pride/shame axis) Conversely, failed intent or inefficacy, if occurring in the context of activation of interest–excitement or joy, may result in a primitive shame reaction. It is a subtle but important distinction whether it is the inefficacy in relation to the environment (especially the human environment) that activates shame or whether it is a barrier to interest–excitement that activates shame, as Tomkins suggests. I opt for the former view, partly for the reason given in Chapter 2—that there are many instances of blocked interest-excitement that are not shame-producing—but also because linking shame to failed intent and inefficacy ties shame to the sense of self and better explains the close relationship between shame and self-feeling.

For the infants in the aforementioned contingency studies, the sense of self was clearly "on the line," and the failed intent, with its associated deflation of interest–excitement and enjoyment, activated shame. It is important to note, however, that these laboratory studies were "artificial" in that they presented the infant with "bizarre" contingency experiences, that in the ordinary and natural course of events would not occur. For the average infant, significant contingency experiences would only occur in interaction with another person. The shame reactions of these infants could have resulted from the infants' generalization of innately interpersonal affective meanings to the non-personal environment.

The possibility that the innate affect of shame could appear early in the first year of life was not considered in most of the earlier literature on shame. Tomkins (1963) was, to my knowledge, the first to suggest that shame/shyness may appear when the infant is able to distinguish the mother's face from the face of a stranger. Izard (1977), in reviewing Tomkins's ideas writes:

> Many people have had the experience of seeing someone in a crowd and eagerly trying to greet and communicate with the individual only to find suddenly that the person whose attention has been claimed is a total stranger. The shame experienced in such a situation may be mild, or intense,

30

depending upon the circumstances. Since an unanticipated friend–stranger differential can elicit shame, Tomkins hypothesizes that as soon as the infant learns to differentiate the face of the mother from the face of the stranger (sometime around the fourth month of life) the infant is vulnerable to shame. (p. 395)

In an earlier publication on shame (1982) I suggested that if Tomkins were right, then it seemed likely that shame could also arise in the infant's interaction with mother at those moments when mother becomes a "stranger" to her infant. That a mother, even a "good enough" mother (to use Winnicott's apt term), could at times be a stranger to her own infant is not so surprising, since the mother's shifting moods, preoccupations, conflicts, and defenses will alter her physiognomy and established communication patterns. The "still face" experiments of Tronick, Als, Adamson, Wise, and Brazelton (1978) seem to provide evidence for this hypothesis. In those experiments interchanges between infants and their mothers were filmed under two different conditions. In the first phase of the experiment, mother was told to interact with her 3-month-old infant as she normally would in a face-to-face exchange. Next, she was instructed to leave the room for a few minutes and upon her return to make eye contact with her infant but not to engage in affective or verbal interaction. When presented with the still-faced mother, for a while the infants would attempt to engage the mother in their usual mode of interaction. When this failed the infants exhibited one of two characteristic behaviors; some cried in distress and others slumped in their seats with a sudden loss of body tonus, turning the head downward and to the side, averting their gaze from the mother's face. Nathanson (1987b), in his discussion of these experiments, concluded that this latter group of infants was exhibiting a shame response.

As I also said in my earlier study of shame, so-called stranger anxiety is at least as much a matter of shame/shyness as it is of anxiety. In support of this idea Nathanson (1987b) cited the following passage in which psychoanalyst and infant researcher Spitz (1965) described the reaction to strangers of the 6- to 8-month-old infant:

31

> If a stranger approaches him, this will release an unmistak-
> able, characteristic and typical behavior in the child; he
> shows varying intensities of apprehension or anxiety and
> rejects the stranger . . . he may lower his eyes "shyly," he
> may cover them with his hands, lift his dress to cover the
> face, throw himself prone on the cot and hide his face in the
> blankets, he may weep or scream. The common denomina-
> tor is a refusal of contact, a turning away, with a shading
> more or less of anxiety. . . . I have called this pattern the
> *eight-month anxiety* and consider it the earliest manifestation
> of *anxiety proper*. (p. 150)

As Nathanson (1987b) pointed out in his discussion of this
passage, "Unless one is burdened by a theory that says shame
cannot appear for another year or so, it is difficult to conceptualize shyness, lowered eyes, and the (pathognomonic for shame)
action of hiding the face as anything but shame" (p. 7).

THE ROLE OF THE OTHER IN THE
DEVELOPMENT OF THE SENSE OF SELF

Shame experiences in infancy represent more or less pure affect
states without the cognition about the self that is characteristic
of shame somewhat later in development. This is because objective self-awareness has not yet been acquired and a concept of
self has not yet been formed. A "sense of self" is present soon
after birth, however, and is founded on efficacy experience and
primary communion with the caretaking other. Since it is the
primary caretaker's responsibility to support the infant's excitement and intentionality, promote a sense of efficacy, and protect
the infant from too many experiences of being unable to influence, comprehend, or predict what transpires in their relationship, early shame experiences frequently represent maternal failure of one kind or another and such experiences weaken the
developing sense of self.

Zaner (1981) refers to the sense of self as essentially depending on "an orientation to an other whose otherness is
disclosed precisely as 'experiencing' the self . . . without that
'making a difference to' . . . it would not be possible for self to

be 'awakened'" (p. 190). The sense of self and sense of other (the other who takes account of me and for whom I make a difference) are thus inseparably linked both in early development and on into maturity.

Trevarthen (1979) insists that there are three inseparable aspects to consciousness: (1) intentionality, knowing what one is doing and why; (2) awareness of the here and now reality, that is, knowing what is being seen, heard, touched, and so forth; and (3) the sharing of knowledge and personal feelings, having intimacy with the consciousness of others and an awareness of affectional and moral responsibility to them. Trevarthen adds that "philosophical investigations often reject one or two of them. The empiricists, for example, have little interest in (1) or (3), yet these two aspects have great importance in every free manifestation of human life where the benefits of consciousness are most obvious" (p. 189). The empiricists, to the extent that they would recognize intentionality and shared consciousness at all, would most likely see them as derived from sensory awareness. These three aspects of consciousness are actually quite interdependent. The traditional empirical view is to assign primacy to awareness of sense data and to view intentionality and shared consciousness as emerging from and subsequent to that sensory awareness. In actuality it is only by virtue of the kinesthetic flows that flesh out rudimentary intentionality that sense data take on organizational significance and meaning in the first place. The infant makes "sense" out of sense data only to the extent that such data are functionally correlated with the kinesthetic flows that serve intentionality and shared consciousness. Trevarthen (1979) makes a similar point when he says, "Perception is not decided by the useful resources of stimulation alone: it requires an approach by the subject's mind, a latent purpose or proposition in relation to which the stimulus affords a setting for activity" (p. 193).

If intentional expression or intimacy with the consciousness of others is disturbed, then there will be some co-disturbance in the awareness of the here-and-now reality, that is, knowing what is being seen heard, touched, and so forth. Understanding these interrelationships has important implications for understanding the nature of what clinicians call "reality testing" and for understanding its possible disturbances.

33

Intentionality and shared consciousness are closely linked with the affect system. Intentionality is "animated by regulatory states of excitement" (Trevarthen, 1979, p. 189). In infancy and early childhood shared consciousness is primarily founded on shared affective meanings and experiences, and such meanings and experiences continue to constitute the core of shared consciousness throughout life. Shame signals a disruption in intentionality and shared consciousness and thus in the sense of self. If Trevarthen is correct, as I believe he is, in asserting that intimacy with the consciousness of others and awareness of our moral and affectional responsibility to them is one of the three innate aspects of consciousness, then one need not postulate a distinct intrapsychic structure, the Freudian superego, to perform that function of regulating our moral and affectional responsibilities toward others.

Trevarthen (1974) concluded from his studies on infant–mother interaction that "the endowment of the human infant for intersubjective functions is greater than that for the transactions of consciousness with the physical nonliving world and [we] would ascribe great theoretical significance to this fact" (p. 185).

The philosopher Scheler (1970) made the observation that

> in the history of philosophy the existence of a real external world has been far more frequently denied than the existence of other selves: and this though no one has denied our ability to perceive Nature, while practically everybody has disputed our power of perceiving mental life in others. The reason for this is that *our conviction of the existence of other minds is earlier and deeper than our belief in the existence of nature.* (p. 259)

We know from the infancy studies of the last two decades that the infant comes into the world well equipped for social interaction on the gestural and affective level. Other persons and their expressions have an uncontested primacy as far as the infant's attention and interest are concerned. Scheler intuitively understood this in 1912. Expression, he said, is the first thing that the infant grasps of the world about him and all sensory experience is initially construed as expressions of mind. It is only in the course of development that the child learns to de-animate a large segment of the world so that ultimately "only a proportion of sensory appearances retains its function as vehicles of expression" (p. 239).

SEEING AND BEING SEEN

The Irish philosopher Bishop Berkeley formulated an idealistic philosophy encapsulated in the famous slogan "*esse est percipi*" (to be is to be perceived). The question of whether objects thus cease to be when there is no one around to perceive them was dealt with by Berkeley through introducing God as the ever-present perceiver, maintaining the existence of objects when no human perceivers were around. This was nicely summarized in the following limerick (cited by Margenau, 1984), presumably composed by some student at Oxford, where Berkeley ended his career.

> *There was a young man who said "God,*
> *to you it must seem very odd*
> > *that a tree as a tree*
> > *simply ceases to be*
> *When there's no one about in the quad."*

God answers:

> *"Young man, your astonishment's odd,*
> *I'm always about in the quad*
> > *and that's why the tree*
> > *never ceases to be*
> *as observed by, yours faithfully, God"*

Berkeley, of course, was dealing with the issue of the existence of the external world. I would like to suggest that Berkeley's famous maxim "*esse est percipi*" could be applied to the problem of the existence and formation of the sense of self. To be perceived by the other and to perceive that one is perceived by the other (which is confirmed by the response of the other to one's

35

gestures and initiations) supports intentionality, establishes a sense of efficacy, and calls into being the sense of self. The sense of self emerges in what Zaner (1981) called "the contextural embrace of other selves."

In this matter of being perceived and perceiving that one is perceived, the sensory modality that carries the heaviest load is sight; thus, seeing and seeing that one is being seen play leading roles in the normal development of the sense of self. (Presumably, other sensory modalities such as hearing and touch would play the leading role in the case of blind infants.) The gaze of the mother and her facial display may be a response to the infant's affective communications or they may contain no response (as in the still-face experiments of Tronick mentioned earlier). The still-face gaze is the prototype of what will become the objectifying gaze, the gaze that denies or ignores one as a subject or self and recognizes only one's surface behavior or material aspects.

The role that seeing and being seen plays in the development of the sense of self now comes together with what we have said earlier about shame. If early shame reflects failed intentionality and failed efficacy vis-à-vis the human environment with concomitant disruption of the positive affects of interest–excitement, enjoyment or joy, then the gaze of the other is apt to be the medium through which this failure is grasped. This could provide the explanation for the abiding association between shame and the wish to hide or avoid the gaze of the other. Seeing and being seen will take on new dimensions of meaning once objective self-awareness is firmly acquired, and it is to that subject we now turn.

·4·

Shame and Objective Self-Awareness

In the previous chapter I suggested that the earliest sense of self was based on, and emergent from, the infant's experience of efficacy, fulfilled intentionality, and the joy and excitement attendant on that experience, all of which takes place in the context of intersubjectivity or shared consciousness. The sense of self is self-consciousness of an immediate, preconceptual, and non-imagistic type; it is the basis of our most profound identification with our body, and it is what provides us with the experience of "indwelling," the experience of the "lived body" rather than the body as part of the object world.

It is the developmental emergence of objective self-awareness that begins to split our experience of ourselves into the public and the immediate or private mode. To be in the "public mode" is to be in the state of objective self-awareness. By objective self-awareness I mean an awareness of oneself as an object for others and, through the mirroring of the observing others, taking oneself as an object of reflection (objectifying oneself). (The reader should note that the word *objective* as used in this work carries no implication of being unbiased or unprejudiced, as it often does.)

The mediation of the other is essential in the foundation of self-objectification. The acquisition of objective self-awareness requires that the child grasp that he is visible to others in the same way that others are visible to him, that is, that he has an

37

exterior on which others can have a perspective *that he can never share*, except in a very limited fashion. The appearance of the capacity for self-objectification is marked by the child's recognition of the image in the mirror as his own, and the *consolidation* of objective self-awareness is marked by the consistently accurate use of personal pronouns. Sharpless (1985) says that "in acquiring person pronouns the child indicates an awareness that he is capable of assuming different perspectives on a situation and that he knows that others may also" (p. 879). For example, the child must grasp that the person pronouns "I" and "me" refer to the speaker whether that speaker be himself or another.

According to Lichtenstein (1963), the subjective sense of self and self-objectification are

> mutually incompatible as psychological experience, i.e., that they really cannot be simultaneously conscious in the same individual. [Thus] the dilemma of human identity . . . centers around self-objectivation versus the subjective experience of the 'actuality of being.' Because I believe that these two ways of experiencing one's identity are mutually exclusive, i.e., man loses the one when he is experiencing the other, I am speaking of the dilemma of human identity. (p. 193)

From the moment the child recognizes the image in the mirror as his own, the body begins to become transformed from a kinesthetic, instrumental presence to a visible presence; at the same time, a transformation of personality begins. The phenomenologist Merleau-Ponty (1964) described the child as learning at this stage that "he is not only what he believed he was by inner experience but he is in addition that figure he sees in the mirror" (p. 153). Merleau-Ponty goes on to say that the look of others also tells me, as does the mirror, that I am limited to a point in space and "that I am that visible 'stand-in' [*doublure*] in whom I would recognize only with difficulty the lived me" (p. 153). As Sardello (1974) points out in his review of Merleau-Ponty's (1964) work, when one begins to realize that one can be seen by others, in an objective sense, there is a tearing of the self from itself; the consequences are that, first, one begins to live an ideal image of oneself and, second, a reflexive relationship with oneself becomes possible. This beginning of a possible relationship with oneself is also the beginning of a kind of alienation from oneself. With the advent of objective self-awareness the child no longer experiences himself as centered in the way he previously felt himself to be or grounded in the previously taken for granted intersubjectivity.

Merleau-Ponty writes,

> The ego, the I, cannot truly emerge at the age of three years without doubling itself with an *ego in the eyes of the other*. In the case of this phenomenon it is not a question of shame, *in the sense in which it exists later on* as the shame of being naked (which appears only around the age of five or six), any more than it is a fear of being reprimanded. It is simply a question of the fear experienced by the child when he is looked at. (p. 153, emphasis mine)

I agree with Merleau-Ponty that the shame that is associated with the acquisition of objective self-awareness is not a matter of shame *as it exists later on*, such as shame about nakedness, but I believe that the child's fear of being looked at is a manifestation of shame anxiety nevertheless. If one holds the view that shame about nakedness marks the earliest appearance of shame (as Merleau-Ponty appears to do), then one would understandably be unlikely to view the 3-year-old child's fear of being looked at as a form of shame anxiety.

For Sartre (1956) shame was not so much a matter of being defective or unworthy but of being an object.

> Shame is the feeling of an original fall not because of the fact that I may have committed this or that particular fault but simply that I have 'fallen' into the world in the midst of things and that I need the mediation of others in order to be what I am. (p. 384)

Shame frequently has to do with experiencing oneself being treated as an object when one is attempting to relate to the other in a intersubjective mode (and conversely, in certain cases, shame may be elicited when one is responded to in a subjective mode when one is presenting oneself as an object—as, for example, when undergoing a physical exam). Recall Schneider's (1977) statement: "we experience shame when we feel we are placed out of the context within which we wish to be interpreted." After the acquisition of objective self-awareness the child may either experience being looked at by the other in a way that supports his intentionality, excitement, and indwelling sense of self or he may experience being looked at in a way that objectifies him and activates shame. Kohut's concept of healthy "mirroring" is consistent with the former type of looking and being looked at. Objectification, on the other hand, could be likened to the look of the camera, which, for Owen Barfield (1977), is the leading symbol of post-Renaissance man because it "looks always at and never into what it sees." Barfield ruefully adds, "I suspect that Medusa did very much the same" (p. 73). For consciousness dominated by objectification, things are opaque, all surface and exterior; one cannot see beyond or through them to what lies on the other side of their surface appearance; things lose their function as clues pointing to something beyond themselves.

Objectification may activate shame because as Lichtenstein has pointed out, self-objectification is incompatible with the actuality of being, the immediate sense of self as indwelling, "connected" to others, and making a difference to those others. If one is relating to the other from this connected, indwelling sense of self and then one suddenly feels objectified, one's sense of self is disturbed and one feels placed out of context. Shame is likely to follow.

In the state of sudden, unsought, or undesired self-objectification the immediate experience of one's actuality of being may be lost, resulting in shame and a disorienting transformation of the interpersonal and phenomenal world. At such times one's world may seem in danger of collapsing. It is as if the ground under one's feet were giving way; depth and spatial relationships may seem altered and one's "place" in space uncertain, resulting in a kind of vertigo. Such experiences dramatically illustrate to what extent the reality of our everyday phenomenal world is dependent on an intact sense of self and an intact set of interpersonal coordinates and not simply on an intact brain or sensory organs.

Following the acquisition of objective self-awareness the experience of the self becomes inexorably split into the immediate I and the mediated, objectified me, and one's experience of the other is split into the other who relates himself to me in such a way as to maintain my subjective sense of self (and to whom I feel emotionally connected) and the other who objectifies me and becomes a potential source of shame (and whom I, in turn, objectify and disconnect from).

Empirical support for the idea that developing objective self-awareness is a trigger for shame comes from the studies of young children's reactions to their mirror images when they first recognize those images as being of themselves. Amsterdam (1972), in her study of mirror self-image reactions in infants and toddlers before age two, concluded that "every subject who showed recognition behavior also manifested either avoidance or self-consciousness or all three" (p. 304). I think it reasonable to conclude that the avoidance and self-consciousness these children exhibited were shame manifestations.

Earlier we extracted from Lynd's (1958) work four basic elements in the shame experience: (1) exposure to others (but also to ourselves) and unexpectedness, the astonishment of the sudden recognition of hitherto unrecognized aspects of ourselves and our relation to aspects of our world; (2) incongruity, the discrepancy between our immediate experience and what appears to us and others from the "outside"; (3) shaken trust in ourselves and others; and (4) confusion, resulting from the loss of the sense of identity we thought we had. All four of these experiential elements of shame affect can be accounted for as a consequence of the sudden shift from the immediate sense of self to objective self-awareness when that shift is unwanted, involuntary, and unexpected.

When the child learns to objectify himself, he simultaneously acquires the ability to compare himself with others and thus becomes sensitive to his relative smallness, weakness, and lack of competence as compared to parents, older siblings, and most other people. So, in addition to the shame of being forced to view oneself as a delimited, defined thing instead of an unbounded consciousness, there is the added shame of also finding oneself to be a rather inferior sort of thing at that. If one must

41

view oneself and be viewed by others as an object, then what kind of an object one is becomes a matter of some importance. Since it is very difficult (largely impossible) to directly assess oneself as an object, one tries to view oneself through the mirroring gaze of the important others in one's lifespace. Being seen and knowing in what light one is being seen take on enormously magnified importance after the acquisition of objective self-awareness.

The *image* of the self and the *ideal* of the self are both brought into being by objective self-awareness. Merleau-Ponty (1964), in his insightful analysis of the consequences of the child's recognition of his own mirror image, observes that from this experience the child will derive "the possibility of an attitude of self-observation that will develop subsequently in the form of narcissism" (p. 137). The mirror image draws the child away from his immediate reality and directs him toward what he sees and imagines himself to be. This "confiscation" of his immediate self by the self visible in the mirror prefigures the confiscation of the immediate self by the others who look at the child.

Objective self-awareness has a derealizing and a depersonalizing function in that it turns the child away from what he immediately is, in order to direct him toward what he sees and imagines himself to be, or *could be*. The individual is thus transformed from an effective, centered being to a being entranced by an imaginal self or an ideal self; there is a primary dissociation here. Since the self as an object of reflection does not exist before objective self-awareness is established, it makes no sense to speak of narcissism—in the classical mythological sense of a morbid fascination with one's own image (or an excessive focusing on or preoccupation with one's self-image)—prior to the acquisition of objective self-awareness.

Freud (1914) connected narcissism and the formation of the ego-ideal with the function of self-observation when he identified conscience as the psychic agency constantly watching the ego and measuring it by comparison to the ego-ideal. This would imply that neither narcissism nor conscience (or what was later designated as the superego) can appear until objective self-awareness has been acquired. Self-objectification and the shame associated with it form the basis of what will later be designated as conscience. The later appearance of guilt may in part be a defense against earlier shame. Miller (1989), pursuing a comment of Erikson's (1950) that shame is often absorbed by guilt, notes that guilt, although burdening, is associated with a sense of strength whereas shame carries with it a painful sense of weakness and vulnerability. By becoming the one who compulsively orders himself about, the young child begins to display guilt feeling but feels less helpless and less vulnerable to shame. Miller suggests that guilt may protect against views of the self as helplessly deficient and thus protect against shame.

PRIMARY COMMUNION AND OBJECT RELATIONS

For the period prior to the acquisition of objective self-awareness, when there is a sense of self but no objective self and a sense of the other but no objective other, I would propose the term *primary communion* rather than the older psychoanalytic term *primary narcissism*. The concept of primary narcissism presupposed an initially unrelated infant who was driven only by the need to relieve drive tension and who only gradually and reluctantly differentiated self from other. In the light of infancy studies of the last two decades, which reveal the infant coming into the world equipped for social interaction from the outset, the infant's supposed lack of self and other differentiation is no longer tenable. Stern (1983, 1985) has been perhaps the most vocal and persuasive critic of these venerable psychoanalytic assumptions about the infant's earliest mental states (see also Lichtenberg, 1983).

We must be careful that in rejecting the idea of primary narcissism we do not naively assume that because the infant recognizes and interacts with the other in an affectively lively way that the other is an "object" to the infant. The word *object* originally meant "something thrown in the way." Somewhere along the way people became "objects" and "part objects" in the theoretical and clinical language of psychoanalysis. The other as "object" in psychoanalytic theory was a necessary and inevitable corollary of drive theory, which assumed a fundamentally sepa-

43

rate, encapsulated, initially unrelated organism who found others of interest only to the degree that they served as suitable "objects" for instinctual drive discharge.

Objecthood is a special status that self and other acquire with the advent of objective self-awareness. Primary communion is a relationship but not an "object" relationship. Since neither the self nor the other exist as objects prior to objective self awareness, object relations precipitate out of primary communion at precisely the time when objective self-awareness is acquired. At a deep experiential level object relations represent a degenerative development—a shameful matter. Sartre (1956) said, "the reaction to shame will consist exactly in apprehending as an object the one who apprehends my own object state" (p. 384). In other words, the moment one becomes an object for oneself, the other also becomes an object. Primary communion is the world of relation established by the primary word I–Thou, to use Martin Buber's (1958) terminology. When one recognizes oneself as an object for the other and feels expelled from the I–Thou, shame is apt to be evoked and one is apt to respond with an objectification of the other, moving into I–It. Farber (1976) writes that Buber

> believed that human experience begins, both in the child and the race, with relation. And, as I have already suggested, what he means by relation may be quite the opposite of what a psychiatrist means by the same word. For a relation imagined from the inside, as a mutual experience, is not the same as an abstract concept of relationship. The latter is "seen" or imagined from the outside, as an event occurring between two human objects. (p. 141)

The loss of primary communion and the shame attendant on that loss become cognitively represented as a "fault." The *Random House Dictionary* defines *fault* as "a defect or imperfection; flaw; failing" and offers a specialized geological meaning of fault: "a break in the continuity of a body of rock or of a vein, with dislocation along the plane of fracture." The loss of primary communion is a fault in a "psychogeological" sense, with psychic dislocation along the plane of fracture; this in turn gives rise to the sense of fault as defect or imperfection in both self and other. To repair that fault then becomes the life project, and the formation of the ideal self and ideal other are the products of that reparative effort. At the heart of the shame experience that follows upon the acquisition of objective self-awareness is the longing for the reestablishment of primary communion; shame becomes nostalgic.

There has been a tendency in psychoanalytic theorizing to confuse the advent of objective self-awareness with self–other differentiation and to assume that, prior to objective self-aware-ness, there is a lack of self–other differentiation. I would say that prior to objective self-awareness, *from the viewpoint of the external observer,* there is no evidence that the infant confuses himself with the other; *from the viewpoint of the infant,* categories having to do with oneness or twoness do not apply because the infant is in the realm of predualistic experience. This does not mean that *experientially* there is a lack of self–other differentiation of a sort but only that *conceptually* there is such a lack. The concept of fusion is dualistic in that it requires the complementary concept of separateness in order to have any meaning; it is a bipolar concept. Dualistic thought requires that what is not separate is fused; however, the rules of dualistic thought are not relevant to the experience of the infant. Therefore, if one asks the question, Does the infant experience himself as one with the caretaking other or as separate? *"both* and *neither"* is as close as one can come to a verbal answer. One is asking a question that is mean-ingless within the predualistic, experiential world of the infant. Thus, the question could well serve as a koan, and some modern day Zen Master might hit one with a stick if one asked it.

SUMMARY

To sum up what we have presented thus far, the acquisition of objective self-awareness is the condition for the emergence of many closely related developments: (1) a heightened vulnerabil-ity to shame affect; (2) the division of experience into the imme-diate and public modes; (3) the split of the self into the imme-diate "I" and the mediated "me"; (4) the loss of primary communion, the original I–Thou; (5) the beginning of "object

45

relations"; (6) the formation of the ideal self and ideal other; (7) the beginnings of conscience; and (8) the birth of narcissism.

SUBJECT OR OBJECT?

The reader at this point might raise the question, Are we not always objects for others in that we have a body and what others see and react to is that body and the behavior of that body? Aren't we always being objectified by others; and if shame is related to objectification, shouldn't we all be in a more or less permanent state of shame? Our response to such questions could only be that of course, in a sense, we are always objects for others but we hope that we are *more* than that. Before the acquisition of objective self-awareness, if we receive healthy parental responsiveness, we exist as pure subjects. After we become aware of ourselves as objects for others we hope that the other will at least regard us as "SUBJECT–objects," that is, that the "subject" aspect of our dual nature for the other will be primary in the other's response to us, thus affirming that we exist together with the other in a field of shared affective experience and overlapping consciousness rather than as disjunctive consciousnesses, surveying each other as mere objects. The parent as mirror must reflect the child as both subject and object so that the child accepts this dual nature of his being for the other; but the emphasis must be on the child as subject, and this emphasis I shall represent by using capitals when writing the term "SUBJECT–object."

I would reserve the term "objectification" for those instances in which the self or the other is not a SUBJECT–object but a subject–OBJECT or mere object. Such objectifications may be subtle or egregious, and rare, recurrent, or continuous. Farber (1976) writes,

> In our ordinary life, in private, we experience one another—
> and our relation—and this is not essentially a visual process.
> We are presences rather than appearances to each other; we
> "read" each other's visible and objective surfaces as a code
> to the more substantial invisibilities—of meaning texture

and habit—of our life together. However that other public form of perception . . . also belongs to us in our private and public worlds. And we feel it most sharply when acquaintances enter our domestic world and we leave it to visit theirs. On such public occasions we fall into experiencing our mates as we imagine they will be experienced by others. Stripped of our private relation, which changes everything, I now see my wife as I think others see her, which is to say that I see her as an aesthetic or sexual or social object. Mannerisms of phrase, countenance, voice, gesture, which usually are no more conspicuous than old prints that have long since merged into the anonymity of the dining-room wall, are now in this new objectivity, brightly lighted and rigorously framed. (pp. 160–161)

This passage illustrates the shifts that may occur in the course of our lives in the way we view one another; from SUBJECT-objects to subject–OBJECTS or even, sadly, to objects.

It is when one is trying to relate to the other as a subject but feels objectified that one is apt to experience shame. A small child approaches his mother excitedly wanting to tell her about something he has just experienced. Mother looks at him and says with a frown, "Your shirttail is hanging out" and proceeds to tuck it in before attending to his communication. The child lowers his head in shame. Tomkins (1963, 1987) and Nathanson (1987b) would interpret the activation of shame affect in this instance as due to the impediment to the child's interest and excitement, but I would put the emphasis on the objectification involved. Such shame-inducing objectifications, although seemingly trivial, if frequent enough lead to a growing insecurity on the child's part as to how he will be responded to—as a SUBJECT-object, a subject–OBJECT, or an object. He develops significant shame anxiety and this anxiety about possibly finding himself a mere object for the other instead of a SUBJECT-object may increase his fear of being looked at. If such objectifications are standard fare for the developing child rather than occasional happenings, the stage is set for the development of significant psychopathology, even possible psychosis. To be continually objectified by the significant other is to have one's very sense of self negated or expropriated by the other. Roustang (1986) talks about the psychotic experience of expropriation.

47

The psychotic does not think, still less does he think of himself: he is produced by thought, he is pure fate, he is not a subject. . . . As an entity, he has been expropriated, and all the thoughts that are properly his own, those that are linked to his perceptions and memories, will bear the stamp of unreality, because there is no subject to which they could be appropriated, unless it is a subject that has itself been expropriated and marked by unreality, without a place of its own, without status, and without recognition. He drifts. If something happens to him, he is the theater in which it happens, but he is not the actor. (p. 133)

The child may either experience the gaze of the other as supporting his intentionality, excitement, and indwelling sense of self, or he may experience being looked at in a way that objectifies him and activates shame. The former way of being looked at leads to the acceptance of oneself as a SUBJECT–object for the other and is consistent with Kohut's concept of healthy mirroring.

If one has not received adequate mirroring from the important caretaking others in one's early life, one's experience of oneself as a SUBJECT–object for the other is unsatisfactory and may lead to efforts to be only subject or only object. Kunkel (1931) made the observation that much human suffering derives from the efforts of individuals to evade the necessity of being both subject and object in our exchanges with one another by trying to be either subject only or object only. According to Kunkel, an individual must, if he is to lead a fully responsible life, accept being both subject and object and thus confront what Lichtenstein called the dilemma of human identity. As Kunkel puts it,

"He may either try to be subject only, confront the world as unhampered and freed from cause and suffering, and withdraw from the responsibility for the results of his action (for being object); or he may try to be object exclusively, to exist merely as a thing without freedom and responsibility, in order thus to escape the discomforts of the living interaction of being subject and object. (pp. 19–20)

Kunkel goes on to point out that the one who tries to be subject only may become the disinterested critic, the inactive onlooker, or perhaps an artist, philosopher, or psychoanalyst. "He will sit on the bank and pretend he is god of the stream, for if he should swim along with the current he would notice far too plainly that it is not he who commands the stream, but the stream him" (p. 21). He who tries to escape the dilemma by being only object may manifest an exaggerated affirmation and compliance with external directives. According to Kunkel, such a person is "the unresisting executor of every foreign will."

Kinston (1983) has presented a theory of shame that stripped of the daunting jargon in which it is wrapped says (if I understand him) that shame occurs when one is tempted to abandon one's authentic subjectivity and become an object, which would lead to one's behavior becoming reactive and mechanical with a loss of spontaneity and autonomy. Whatever the merits of Kinston's theory, he does seem to recognize the importance of the subject or object dilemma in understanding shame.

In a later chapter we see how electing to assiduously devote oneself to being an object may paradoxically be used in an attempt to eliminate the shame of objectification. First, however, we take a closer look at the relationship between shame and narcissism.

·5·

Shame and Narcissism

The importance of the individual's struggles with his shame, the incessant effort to vanquish or come to terms with the alienating affect, his surrenders, transient or chronic, have too often been disregarded by personality theorists in their quest for a static structure which will describe a personality.

SILVAN TOMKINS

In a footnote to Freud's (1914) paper "On Narcissism: An Introduction," it is mentioned that Havelock Ellis in 1898 first used the term "narcissus-like" as a description of a psychological attitude and that Paul Nacke in 1899 introduced the term *narcissism* to refer to a sexual perversion in which the individual takes his own body as the primary object of sexual interest. Freud borrowed the term from Nacke and used it not to refer to a sexual perversion but to "the libidinal complement to the egoism of the instinct of self preservation, a measure of which may justifiably be attributed to every living creature" (p. 74). Thus the notion of "normal" narcissism was born.

Interwoven in Freud's ideas about narcissism are clinical and metapsychological concepts; they are not always very clearly differentiated. Clinical concepts are those that are more experience-near and tied more closely to clinical observation; metapsychological concepts are more abstract and "explanatory" in a grand, theoretical way.

51

On the metapsychological level Freud postulated a line of development for the sexual instinct in which the energy of that instinct, the libido, progressed from a state of autoerotism, prior to the emergence of the ego, to primary narcissism (when libido is entirely directed toward the ego—the first love object), to object love (homosexual and heterosexual). Libido may be subsequently withdrawn from objects and reinvested in the ego, leading to the state of secondary narcissism. In "The Ego and the Id" Freud contradicted this earlier notion of primary narcissism (presented in the 1914 narcissism paper) when he wrote that objects were first "cathected" with libido and that only after the ego had grown strong enough to force itself on the id as a love object did the ego become the focus of the libido.

Freud advanced the idea that in pathological narcissism one's own ego is the more or less exclusive love object, and consequently, there is an impaired capacity for object love. If there is a fixed, limited supply of libido (*libido* and *love* are used interchangeably in Freud's discussion), then the more libido is directed toward others the more impoverished the ego becomes and vice versa. Freud (1914) equates narcissistic depletion of the ego with lowered self-regard. "A person who loves has, so to speak, forfeited a part of his narcissism, and it can only be replaced by his being loved" (p. 98). This is a very curious statement. It suggests that our love of others results in our own ego depletion, lowering our self-regard, and conversely, that the other's ego depletion (in loving us) becomes our ego enrichment. If this is so, then the deployment of libido becomes not strictly an intrapsychic process but an interpersonal one— quantities of libido can apparently be transferred from one psyche to another; lowered self-regard becomes a matter of a trade deficit, as it were.

The actual key to the relationship between some forms of love and lowered self-regard is contained in another statement that Freud (1914) makes in the narcissism paper. He says, "Loving in itself, *insofar as it involves longing and deprivation*, lowers self-regard; whereas being loved, having one's love returned, and possessing the loved object, raises it once more" (p. 99, emphasis mine). The key to understanding this state of affairs is the fact that shame is a universal reaction to unrequited romantic love, as

52

Lewis (1971) noted. The lowered self-regard in this case is a shame manifestation. Forms of love that don't involve "longing and deprivation" because they don't demand reciprocation don't lower self-regard but enhance it, as everyday experience confirms.

It is not my intent to present a thorough critique of Freud's ideas about narcissism or to attempt a thorough review of the literature on narcissism but, rather, to focus on the relationship between shame and narcissism. The term *narcissism* is bandied about in clinical and social discussions in such a loose way that many people feel its usefulness has been seriously compromised and we might do better to abandon the term. *Narcissism* is often used simply to designate any form of self-love. Or the term may be used to refer to a highly inflated sense of one's own importance, in which excessive self-reference testifies to that bloated self-estimate. When clinicians talk about pathological narcissism, implied is an inability to care about others in their own right (and a tendency to use others in an exploitive way in the service of one's own self-aggrandizement) and/or an inability to put oneself in the other's position or critically appraise oneself from the other's point of view. Relationships with others are characterized by a tacit attitude that Balint (1968) formulated as follows:

> It is only my own wishes, interests and needs that matter: none of the people who are important to me must have any interests, wishes, needs different from mine, and if they have any at all, they must subordinate theirs to mine without any resentment or strain; in fact, it must be their pleasure and their enjoyment to fit in with my wishes. (pp. 70–71)

Most everyone would agree that such an attitude toward others is normal for the young child but undesirable in an older person. Respect for the true "otherness" of the other is obviously a developmental achievement and not something we are born with. The other as SUBJECT–object does not exist for the pathological narcissist. He can only treat the other as object, or subject–OBJECT at best. It is not only the other whom the narcissist objectifies, it is himself as well. His own subjectivity is sacrificed to his object self.

53

It is possible to understand narcissism in a way that is faithful to the myth of Narcissus, a youth who became totally absorbed with his own reflection at the expense of interest in the others and the world, and therefore I use the term to denote a disturbance in the self-image that results in an excessive expenditure of energy, attention, and concern to maintain or bolster that deviant self-image. One might ask, How does one determine the proper amount of attention to be paid to one's self-image? My answer would be "with great difficulty." Isn't that one of the most vexing questions every person struggles with (unless he is *so* narcissistic the question never occurs to him)? I'm reminded of one wag's definition of an alcoholic as "someone who drinks more than I do." Similarly, one could say that a narcissist is someone who is more self-preoccupied than I am. Although my comment is obviously facetious, it points up the somewhat arbitrary, subjective nature of many clinical judgements, something that is unavoidable. How outgoing and externally focused does one have to be to qualify as an extrovert? How exuberant and elated does one have to be, and for how long, to be considered hypomanic? In our everyday work we use a host of personality designations that are never precisely quantifiable; why should it be different with narcissism? Although I am sympathetic to the frustration of those who feel the term is abused and ought to be discarded, I don't think the term will disappear so easily and therefore we need to persist in trying to arrive at some consensus as to its proper use.

Before elaborating on my own efforts to arrive at a better understanding of narcissism, I would like to review Morrison's (1989) recent work on the relationship between shame and narcissism, since there are many areas of close agreement between his views and my own. Morrison has been one of the principal contributors to recent psychoanalytic literature on shame, particularly the literature on shame and narcissism. Morrison shares my view that the classical psychoanalytic drive-defense (conflict) theory is too limited in scope to adequately account for the relationship between shame, identity, ideals, failure, and the self.

Although unhappy with Kohut's narrow view of the nature of shame, Morrison argues convincingly that it is the language of

54

shame that permeates Kohut's work and that many aspects of shame, particularly the relationship between shame and narcissism, can be better understood using the constructs of self psychology. Morrison weaves into the framework of Kohutian formulations a modified version of Piers's (Piers & Singer, 1953) thesis that shame is reflective of tension between the ego and the ego-ideal. He translates Piers's structural terms into the language of self psychology, resulting in the restatement that shame reflects severe tension or strain between the self and the ideal self.

Morrison goes on to suggest that shame may result not only from failure in attaining the shape of the ideal self but also from the failure of the selfobject to provide adequate mirroring responsiveness for the grandiose self. One implication of this view would seem to be that when one encounters shame in the clinical situation, one must ask, To whose failure is the patient responding with shame, his own failure or that of the other? The enduring experience of shame may reflect the depleted self that has failed to receive adequate responsiveness from the idealized selfobject. Morrison's (1989) view of shame as a response to selfobject failure is consistent with the views I presented earlier—that shame in the young child represents maternal failure in providing adequate mirroring for the child's developing sense of self.

Morrison asks whether the ultimate goal of the self is reunion and merger with the idealized object or autonomy, independence, uniqueness, competence, and perfection. He argues that these aims, although seemingly antithetical, are manifestations of what he calls "the dialectic of narcissism," an expression he uses to refer to the complementary nature of these narcissistic aims and their alternating figure–ground relationship to each other. Does grandiosity beget an inevitable sense of failure and thus generate shame, or does shame beget grandiosity in order to deny and eliminate a sense of failure? Morrison maintains that it works both ways.

Morrison distinguishes between the nature of shame experience in narcissistic disorders and in neurotic conditions. In the former, shame is more central and underlies the self's total subjective experience. In the latter group, says Morrison, shame tends to be more specifically tied to certain types of conflict, often representing a defensive reaction against painful oedipal conflict and aggression.

To present my own views on narcissism, it might be helpful to first review some points made in the last chapter. There I presented the claim that the *idea* of the self and the *ideal* of the self are both brought into being by objective self-awareness. I referred to Merleau-Ponty's (1964) insightful analysis of the consequences of the child's recognition of his own mirror image and his observation that from this experience the child will derive "the possibility of an attitude of self-observation that will develop subsequently in the form of narcissism" (p. 137). The mirror image draws the child away from his immediate reality and directs him toward what he sees and imagines himself to be. This "confiscation" of the immediate I by the visible me in the mirror prefigures the "confiscation" of the immediate I by the others who mirror the me.

Since the self as an object of reflection doesn't exist before objective self-awareness is established, narcissism becomes possible only after objective self-awareness is established. It is important to remember that in the myth Narcissus became entranced not by his self but by his *image*, his reflection. To the extent that one is excessively preoccupied with or dominated by concerns about one's image, one's status, or oneself as an object for others, to that extent one is narcissistic. The other ("internalized" or not) has become the reflecting pool in which one loses oneself—quite literally losing that indwelling sense of self that I discussed earlier. This is the dilemma of identity that Lichtenstein (1963) talked about, namely, that the experience of the actuality of being and self-objectification are mutually incompatible experiences; in gaining one we lose the other.

Another significant difference between the way of conceptualizing narcissism presented here and earlier ideas about narcissism is that in this model it makes no difference whether the emotion one feels for the objectified self is positive or negative. Whether our Narcissus loves or hates his reflected image is beside the point; the point is that he is captured and dominated by it. From this we derive our differentiation between what has been referred to in the literature as "normal narcissism" and "pathological narcissism." In the case of "normal narcissism" one can move freely back and forth between sense of self as dwelling in the lived body and the state of self-objectification. In "pathological narcissism" one has been more thoroughly captured by self-images and the exaggerated concern for how one appears to others and to oneself. One has lost the unself-conscious sense of self with its possibility for recovering primary communion with the world and its ability to dissolve, at the affective level, the sense of distance and alienation from others that is the corollary of self-objectification.

Joffe and Sandler (1967) hypothesize that the basic form of unpleasure in disturbances of narcissism is an affective experience of mental pain that reflects a substantial discrepancy between the mental representation of the actual self at the moment and the ideal shape of the self. They go on to say that "lack of self-esteem, feelings of inferiority and unworthiness, shame, and guilt all represent particular higher order derivatives of the basic affect of pain" (p. 65). As we have already seen, lack of self-esteem and feelings of inferiority and unworthiness are shame variants. By relegating shame to a later derivative position, Joffe and and Sandler fail to consider the possibility that the basic affective experience of mental pain to which they refer is shame itself. When they suggest that this basic mental pain reflects a discrepancy between the mental representations of the actual self of the moment and the ideal self, are they not pointing to the same affect which Piers (Piers & Singer, 1953) saw as resulting from a failure to live up to one's ego-ideal, namely, shame?

In Chapter 2 we advanced the idea that shame experiences in infancy are, to begin with, affect states without cognition about the self. Cognition about the self becomes associated with shame after objective self-awareness had been acquired. With the advent of objective self-awareness, the child becomes acutely conscious of his comparative smallness, weakness, and incompetence vis-à-vis older persons. For the child who arrives at self-objectification with an already weakened sense of self and considerable shame experience, these discoveries of his relative deficiencies in the larger scheme of things will be more apt to overload the child's shame tolerance, necessitating that he undertake various defensive and compensatory maneuvers. Need-

57

less to say, active shaming and humiliation at the hands of parents, siblings, and others will assist in raising shame to toxic levels.

Joffe and Sandler (1967) suggest that the term *ideal self* be used

> to denote the particular shape of the self-representation at any moment in the individual's life which is believed, consciously or unconsciously, to embody the ideal state. . . . The specialized form of ideal which ensues when the child needs to aggrandize himself for the purpose of defense can be referred to as the "idealized self," but it should be borne in mind that idealization is only one possible source of the content of the ideal self. (p. 64)

Although I believe that idealization is always operative in the formation of the ideal self, the child who arrives at objective self-awareness with a weakened sense of self and significant shame experience will have a stronger need to aggrandize himself in the form of what Sandler and Joffe have called the "idealized self." In Kohut's self psychology, which I briefly discussed in Chapter 1, this "idealized self" is labeled the "grandiose self" and its defensive functions are not acknowledged. Grandiosity is taken to be the natural original state of the self along with the need for an idealized selfobject.

Kernberg (1975), contrasting his views on pathological narcissism with those of Kohut, noted a basic disagreement between himself and Kohut regarding the origin of the grandiose self: In Kohut's view it reflected the fixation of an archaic "normal" primitive self, whereas in Kernberg's view, it was a pathological structure, clearly different from normal infantile narcissism. On this issue my position would be closer to Kernberg's, but I would replace his emphasis on envy as the major affect contributing to the psychopathology of narcissism with an emphasis on shame. I regard the development of the idealized self or grandiose self as occurring only after the advent of objective self-awareness and as reflecting greater mental pain (shame) than normal in the developing child. This situation would result in exaggerated compensatory elaborations of a fantastic and grandiose nature in the formation of the ideal self, justifying the label

idealized self or *grandiose self*. (I prefer the term *idealized self* to
grandiose self because the latter term is somewhat deprecatory.) It
should be emphasized, however, that there is no sharp dividing
line between the normal ideal self and the pathological idealized
self. The normal ideal self also has reparatory functions, as we
saw earlier. Shame is the instigating force in the creation of the
idealized self, and the construction of an idealized self always
implies the coexistence of a devalued shame-ridden self, which is
in dynamic interaction with the idealized self.

In the scheme I am proposing for understanding narcissistic
disorders, objective self-awareness leads to the formation of
three sets of self-images, which can be designated the idealized
("grandiose") self, the "realistic" self, and the devalued self. The
"realistic" self, although a product of self-objectification, is a
more balanced representation of one's real assets and liabilities
and is more apt to be consensually validated by unbiased ob-
servers.

These three sets of self-images are not to be analogized to
static representations of an isolated self but, instead, are to be
understood as fantasy systems, that is, as families of imagina-
tively elaborated "scenes." In the case of the idealized self such
scenes might include those in which one is gloriously trium-
phant, heroically successful, extraordinarily competent or sexually attractive, admired by others, and so forth. In the case of the
the devalued self, such scenes would have to do with situations
(remembered or imagined) in which one was depreciated, humiliated, rejected, or scorned.

We may formulate a rough typology of narcissistic disorders based on which self-image is behaviorally more dominant
in the personality functioning of the individual. In an earlier
work (1982), I identified two basic types of narcissist, which I
provisionally designated as the (relatively) unconflicted egotistical type and the dissociative type. I would presently add a third
type. These three types are characterized as follows:

1. When the idealized self is dominant, we see a type of
narcissist who is unabashedly self aggrandizing and seemingly
shameless. This type, which I have designated *the unconflicted
egotistical type* displays a seemingly total lack of tension between

59

the idealized self and the realistic self, and thus there is an apparent absence of shame. It might be more accurate to say that these individuals lack a well-formed, realistic self-representation. Such an individual is selectively inattentive to all negatively toned critical reactions of others; aspects of the disowned and devalued self are apt to be consistently attributed to others. This type of narcissist has won an apparent victory over shame but at the price of impaired interpersonal sensitivity and impaired self-evaluative functions. Such individuals often are reared by "adoring," doting, narcissistically disturbed parents who have objectified the child and through their adoring gaze have projected onto the child aspects of their own idealized self; these parents have not only failed to provide adequate support for the child's true sense of self but have also failed to provide enough realistic positive and negative evaluation to support some degree of tension between the actual self and the idealized self. Never having been really seen in his early development as a SUBJECT–object, this type of narcissist never really sees others as SUBJECT-objects, which gives his relationships their shallow, superficial, often manipulative quality.

2. When the devalued self is dominant in the functioning of the personality, then we have a type that I earlier designated as the *dissociative type*. Low self-esteem, vulnerability to frequent shame experiences, and rejection sensitivity, as well as diminished energy and vitality characterize this type. The idealized self exists in a split-off dissociative form and is often detectable in the form of a subtle air of superiority and entitlement that exists side by side with a more consciously articulated self-devaluation. The dissociated idealized self is frequently sought for and found—through projection—in certain others, leading to a readiness for the idealization of those others.

3. Tomkins (1982, personal communication), reacting to my introductions of the first two types of narcissist, pointed out, and I agree, that the most frequently encountered type would be one characterized by an unstable equilibrium between these self constructions, with violent lability between the self as engulfed by shame, as reaching out to the ideal other, as projecting its shame onto the bad other, as manipulating the other to support the idealized self, as truly admiring the idealized self, and so

forth. Turbulence between these sharply contrasting selves and the scenes in which they are manifest produces confusion and ambiguity for the individual experiencing such rapidly shifting states. Tomkins adds that "this type of organization produces a pluralism of selves and of others and of scenes which defy integration, not because the ego is weak but because it is too fragmented." I designate this third type of narcissist as the *turbulent type*. This type would include many individuals currently labeled as "borderline" personalities.

Gabbard has recently (1989) described two subtypes of narcissistic personality disorder, which he labeled the "oblivious type" and the "hypervigilant type." These subtypes, as Gabbard describes them, appear to be closely related to my egotistical and dissociative subtypes. Gabbard's oblivious type is described as arrogant and aggressive, self-absorbed, and attention demanding. He is insensitive to the reactions of others and impervious to their hurt feelings. He has a "sender" but no "receiver." The hypervigilant narcissist, according to Gabbard, is inhibited, shy, self-effacing, and shuns being the center of attention. He is very sensitive to slights and criticisms and is prone to feeling ashamed or humiliated.

As I noted in my earlier work (1982) on this subject, the discrepancies between Kohut's and Kernberg's views of narcissistic personalities—discrepancies that are usually attributed to different theoretical orientations—appear, to some extent, to reflect a difference in the narcissistic prototypes on which they based their formulations. Gabbard (1989) echoes this point. Kernberg seems to have had the egotistical type as his prototype, and Kohut the dissociative type. The egotistical type is more apt to devalue the analyst or therapist and the dissociative type is more apt to idealize him. I suspect that the countertransference evoked by the patients belonging to the different subtypes may have significantly colored these clinicians' theoretical formulations on narcissistic personalities, which would account for the impression that Kernberg is engaged in "anathematization" more than diagnosis in his characterization of narcissistic personalities, and conversely that Kohut has a much friendlier view.

In the case of what I have called the dissociative type, shame may play a double role—as an instigating force in the construction of the grandiose self and also as the affect responsible for the defensive "splitting off" of the grandiose self from the rest of the self organization. Kohut (1971) writes that the aim of analysis is to bring about "the inclusion into the adult personality (the reality ego) of the repressed or otherwise nonintegrated (isolated, split-off, disavowed) aspects of the grandiose self" (p. 147). This task, says Kohut, proceeds in the face of strong resistances that are "mainly motivated by shame" (p. 154).

Kohut's analytic work with narcissistic personalities consisted, in no small part, of helping the patient to master or mitigate the intense shame that maintained the dissociation, disavowal, or splitting off of the grandiose self, although Kohut himself did not explicitly conceptualize his work in this way. However, Morrison (1983) has pointed out, that although the word "shame" does not appear very frequently in Kohut's writing, "it is the language of shame which permeates his work" (p. 310). Morrison notes Kohut's references to "self-esteem," "disturbed self-acceptance," "dejection of defeat," "defective self," "mortification of being exposed," "guiltless despair," "hopelessness," and "lethargy," as illustrative of the concern with shame implicit in Kohut's writings.

Kernberg's (1975) emphasis on the importance of "splitting" in narcissistic personalities also reflects an insufficient appreciation of the role of shame in the formation and maintenance of what appear to be "split-off" aspects of the personality. Of splitting in an individual with a narcissistic personality disorder, Kernberg says "haughty grandiosity, shyness, and feelings of inferiority may coexist without affecting each other" (p. 265). What Kernberg fails to recognize is that haughty grandiosity, shyness, and feelings of inferiority are all forms of shame or reactions to shame and, as such, are apt to be surrounded by secondary shame. In secondary shame one is ashamed of being ashamed; one may thus be ashamed of such shame manifestations as shyness, grandiosity, and feelings of inferiority. The motive for keeping these aspects of oneself split-off is to avoid the shame that would ensue upon their recognition. What Kernberg labels as "splitting" is simply the normal operation of shame dynamics.

IS PSYCHOANALYSIS
A NARCISSISTIC ENTERPRISE?

James Hillman (1989), in a stimulating article entitled "From Mirror to Window: Curing Psychoanalysis of Its Narcissism" suggests that the current, somewhat faddish interest in narcissism is reflective of some fundamental narcissistic disturbance within depth psychology and psychoanalysis itself. Hillman points out that psychoanalysis (as a movement) idealizes itself, has had an inflated notion of its own power and the importance of its place in history, is enormously invested in watching itself and its practitioners (interminable supervision), and is extremely self-referential, in referring all events back to itself as the frame in which they are to be understood. Hillman refers to the analytic idealization of transference as "that self-gratifying analytical habit which refers the emotions of life to the analysis. Transference habitually deflects object libido, that is, love for anything outside analysis, into a narcissistic reflection on analysis. We feed analysis with life" (p. 65).

According to Hillman, the narcissism of the analytic situation leads to the increasing libidinal importance of the other—analyst for patient and patient for analyst—as the only way out of that narcissism, while at the same time the taboo prohibits their acting on their need for the other. Hillman feels that the desire for cure by love rather than cure by analysis arises not so much from the narcissism of the patient (as Freud implied) as from the narcissism of the analytic system in which the patient is situated. Hillman suggests that if the participants should sometimes act out the love cure fantasy, it may be in reaction to the narcissism of analysis (which grandiosely promises cure in the first place, not in each individual case, but in principle). Hillman says:

> By elaborating ethical codes, malpractice insurance, investigations and expulsions which blame the participants, analysis protects itself from wounding insights about its own narcissism. The vulnerability of analysis—that its effectiveness is always in question, that it is neither science nor

medicine, that it is aging into professional mediocrity and may have lost its soul to power years ago despite its idealized language of growth and creativity (a language, by the way, never used by its founders)—this vulnerability is overcome by idealizing the transference. (p. 66)

The vulnerability that Hillman describes is shame vulnerability, the failure of analysis to measure up to its grandiose self-image. Thus, we are brought back once again to the recurrent link between shame and narcissism.

Although I believe Hillman is making an important observation about psychoanalysis, I am uncomfortable with attributing narcissism to the psychoanalytic situation, method, or movement because, in my view, narcissism can rightly be ascribed only to persons. Activities may be said to be narcissistic only to the extent that they represent the narcissistic concerns of the persons engaged in those activities. I think it more correct to say that the analytic method, with its idealization of the transference and its emphasis on transference analysis, permits the analyst to freely indulge his narcissism. Although the patient may be talking about some interaction in his life outside the analysis, *the analyst listens to find himself in the material.* Were he not engaged in the narcissistically gratifying activity of examining the material for references to himself, he might not be able to listen to patients hour after hour, day after day, with the same quality of attention without drifting into escapist reveries of various kinds.

I view the situation as follows: the analyst is gazing into the reflecting pool of the patient's material to find himself. Although ostensibly he is looking to find himself as transference object, I believe that on a deeper, more unconscious level he often looks in the hope of finding his "true self." Stone (Langs & Stone, 1980) recalled a remark by Glover (Glover, 1937) to the effect that "in the last analysis the patient is searching for and reacts to the kind of person that the analyst really is in the depths of his personality" (Stone, p. 37). I believe that the analyst, like his patient, may be searching for the kind of person he (the analyst) really is which means that often there may be this hidden agenda operating behind the task of analyzing the patient. Looked at in this way, analysis (and much analytic psychotherapy) could be described as an elaborate, unacknowledged game of "hide and seek," in which the analyst hides and both parties then seek to find him.

It has always been of interest to me that most of the major contributors to the clinical literature on the understanding and treatment of the narcissistic personality have been training analysts, people who spend their clinical hours analyzing other analysts (candidates) in training. These candidates, it seems reasonable to assume, are people presumably very much like the training analyst himself in many important ways. If the narcissistic personality is what training analysts are so expert at treating, then one would suspect that narcissism must be rampant in the psychoanalytic institutes and societies. Or is the narcissism with which analysts are so obsessed really a projected form of their own individual and collective narcissism, a narcissism crystallized in analytic theory and technique?

·III·

Interpersonal Dimensions
of Shame

·6·

Shame Imposed
and Inherited

Esteem and disgrace are, of all others, the most powerful incentives to the mind, when once it is brought to relish them. If you can get into children a love of credit, and an apprehension of shame and disgrace, you have put into them the true principle, which will constantly work and incline them to the right.

JOHN LOCKE

THE BLUSH

Because we tend to experience our self as most present in the face, shame having to do with a sense of personal unworthiness is apt to be quite visible in the face, not only in the form of a lowered head and averted gaze but in the form of a blush as well. The experience of shame after objective self-awareness has been acquired is not necessarily accompanied by blushing in all cases. Some shame dominated persons never blush; they may lower their head or avert their gaze in shame but show no visible change in color. Some people pale or become livid when they feel shame. There is undoubtedly a physiological predisposition to blushing.

Feldman (1962) asserts that "in order to blush a person has to be ordered to be ashamed." Blushing may begin as a manifestation of imposed shame and may signal compliance with that imposition. Shame is apt to be imposed by parents or educators with a phrase such as "You should be ashamed of yourself" or "Shame on you." Feldman says that although a stern look might later do the same thing, it is primarily *the word* that underlies the imposition. Wondering how an affect can be imposed upon an individual, Feldman postulates that shame manifested as blushing occurs against a background of preexisting anxiety of not being loved and of being isolated by exclusion. Feldman cites Hermann's (1943) untranslated work to the effect that blushing is the "flowing over" of the flaming look of the other, a form of affect contagion. The parent feels shame over some piece of the child's behavior and immediately attempts to relocate that shame in the child, where, from the parent's view, it properly belongs. The child's compliance in accepting the shame is signaled by the lowered head, averted gaze, and the blush.

The feared separation at this stage is from the group rather than from a single person, according to Hermann. This is, to my way of thinking, a very important observation. It has been my experience that blushing is most frequent in those individuals who have a chronically high level of social anxiety, in other words, in those for whom the issue of social acceptability versus unacceptability is of paramount concern. This chronically high level of social anxiety is often associated with autonomic overactivity and excessive vascular reactivity. The ability of beta-adrenergic blockers to allay performance anxiety (*shame anxiety* would be a more accurate term) and relieve social phobias, including the fear of blushing, testifies to the importance of sympathetic overactivity as a background condition for excessive blushing.

The blushing child has grasped the fact that violation of group norms (not the violation of laws, which would elicit guilt) may result in exclusion or the threat of exclusion, and the loved parent may "betray" (from the child's point of view) and shame the child in obeisance to those group norms. The relevant social field is suddenly and frighteningly enlarged from the dyad to the group. The child is now forced to consider the question, What will people think? and that question may subsequently dominate his life, pushing him into a more or less permanent state of self-objectification. Darwin (1872) wrote, "It is not the simple act of reflecting on our own appearance, but the thinking what others think of us which excites the blush." The importance of the group in the shame experience associated with blushing is confirmed by the fact that even into adulthood blushers are more apt to blush or fear blushing in group situations and are much less likely to blush in one-to-one encounters or when alone.

A female patient, in exploring her readiness to blush, noted that her blushing was more apt to be triggered by a compliment, such as a favorable remark about her appearance from a co-worker, but only if that remark was made in the presence of others. Analysis revealed a fantasy that the compliment would arouse the envy and hostility of the other females present; the blush was in part a signal to her peers that she disavowed the compliment and thus an attempt to appease them and ward off their envy. She feared standing out as too different from others in any way—either positive or negative—for fear of exclusion.

The child's acceptance of imposed shame is signaled by the blush, lowered head, and averted gaze. The blush and lowered head together serve as an appeasement gesture, designed to forestall exclusion and to signal acceptance of the negative judgment of the important others. According to Feldman, blushing may appear as early as the age of 2 to 3 years, when the ego-ideal and superego are in the process of formation. My own impression is that blushing is more apt to appear somewhat later and is apt to be most pronounced in adolescence, owing to the increased importance of peer group acceptance and the upsurge of sexual excitement. Anything that increases sexual arousal also potentially increases shame vulnerability and the tendency to blush, since shame regulates the sexual drive. I will discuss that relationship in more depth later.

HUMILIATION, CONTEMPT, AND BORROWED SHAME

The ubiquity of the experience of humiliation at the hands of our fellow human beings and the toxicity of that experience were painfully noted by Swedish film director Ingmar Bergman (1973):

> One of the strongest feelings I remember from my childhood is precisely of being humiliated; of being knocked about by words, acts or situations. Isn't it a fact children are always feeling deeply humiliated in their relations with grownups and each other? . . . Our whole education is just one long humiliation, and it was even more so when I was a child. One of the wounds I've found hardest to bear in my adult life has been the fear of humiliation and the sense of being humiliated. Every time I read a review, for instance—whether laudatory or not—this feeling awakes . . . to humiliate and be humiliated, I think, is a crucial element in our whole social structure. It's not only the artist I'm sorry for. It's just that I know exactly where he feels most humiliated. Our bureaucracy, for instance. I regard it as in high degree built up on humiliation, one of the nastiest and most dangerous of all poisons. When someone has been humiliated he's sure to try to figure out how the devil he can get his own back, humiliate someone else in turn, until, maybe the other feels so humiliated that he's broken, can't humiliate back again, or doesn't even bother to figure out how he can do so. (pp. 80–81)

Morrison (1989) suggests that contempt may be viewed as the projective identification of shame. Although I regard the concept of projective identification as an oxymoron, I believe that the interpersonal process for which it tries to account is real enough. Morrison maintains that contempt is an attempt to rid the self of shame by an effort to relocate it in another person. The recipient of the projected shame is pressured in various ways to take ownership of the shame and is then treated with disdain and scorn. When the one who projects his shame onto the other remains in ongoing interaction with the recipient of his projection, this is interpreted by some as evidence of a continued "identification" with the projected aspect of the self.

If we accept Morrison's notion that contempt often represents the projective identification of shame, then logically we must also accept that shame often represents the "introjective identification" (one infelicitous term deserves another) of the other's shame, that is, one accepts the shame projected by the other and "identifies" with it and with the other's contempt for the self. It is not uncommon for families to use one child as the repository for the shame of the parents and other family members. The child in that situation can never dare successfully compete with others because the pressures on him to contain the projected feelings of shame and failure for the family are too intense and whatever acceptance or tolerance he enjoys is dependent on his willingness to function in that role.

One may accept the shame of the other as one's own even in the absence of projective identification. It is a fairly common observation that many individuals feel shame over some aspect of their parents' or children's lives (about which the individual himself may or may not feel shame) and experience this shame as though it were their own. I think of this as "borrowed" or inherited shame.

An Example of Borrowed Shame

Alice, a 63-year-old widow, whom I had treated for depression and anxiety some years earlier, returned to see me because of a recurrence of her symptoms. This time she revealed to me information that she had been too ashamed to talk about in our earlier contacts. She had grown up in upstate New York in the 30s and 40s with an alcoholic father who worked as a salesman in his father's car dealership and also sold real estate. When her father collected his commission after a successful real estate transaction, he would usually go off on a drinking binge, during which time he would squander the money he had made.

My patient worked her way through college and after gradu- ation moved to Boston, where her brother lived. He found her a place to live and helped her find a job at the medical school where he taught. This brother later bought a home and arranged for mother and father to come to Boston to live with him and my patient also moved in with them at that time. Father found a job as manager of a local grocery store but continued to drink heavily. Alice worried about bringing friends into the house for fear of being embarrassed by father's drunkenness. Around this time she met her husband-to-be, a medical student, and began dating him. They fell in love and planned to marry.

In the meantime, father ran off to Las Vegas with a woman he worked with in the grocery store. He wrote the patient's mother, asking for a divorce, and she refused. He returned to upstate New York with his girlfriend and tried to find work but without success; his girlfriend also looked for work and one day after a job hunting foray, returned to their apartment to find him dead on the floor with the gas turned on. When the family learned of his death, they conspired to keep his suicide a secret. The patient's brother called a friend on the staff of the local newspaper to ask him to keep the circumstances of father's death out of the paper; the friend obliged.

My patient feared that if her fiancé found out about her father's suicide, he mighty change his mind about marrying her. She struggled with how to tell him—and even whether she should tell him. Before she could resolve her internal struggle, her fiancé one day came to her and told her that he had some information to share with her, information that was very difficult for him to share but that he felt she needed to know before they married. Anxious and alarmed, she nevertheless urged him to confide in her. With obvious signs of struggle he then confessed that his father had committed suicide. Far from being upset by this revelation, my patient was greatly relieved, for now she could confess that her own father had also committed suicide. Their shame became a shared shame. After they married they conspired to keep this information from their children and were able to do so for many years until a distant relative revealed it to one of the children, an event that humiliated and infuriated my patient.

This secret of her father's suicide had haunted my patient's life; the borrowed shame of it was a significant factor predisposing her to depressive episodes. That she could have undergone previous treatment while concealing this significant information was a testimony to the depth of her shame. One might argue that some of the shame, which in her mind was attached to her father's alcoholism and suicide may have sprung from other sources in her psychosexual development. Although this may have been true, it was not necessary to pursue other

74

sources of shame in order to bring about a significant clinical improvement. The confession and reevaluation of her shame were enough.

SOURCES OF SHAME

The variety of possible sources of shame makes it difficult for the individual to correctly identify the actual source of enduring shame in his self-experience. Is the chronic shame he feels the result of his own failure or the failure of significant others to provide affirmation that he is a SUBJECT–object for them, or is it the pressured acceptance of the other's projected shame, or is it borrowed or inherited shame? Or is it the result of some combination of these sources? Unfortunately, shame often becomes a central aspect of the child's core self-experience before he has the cognitive ability to even begin to sort out and identify the sources of his shame.

Contempt for others will usually go hand in hand with the desire or willingness to humiliate them. *The Random House Dictionary* indicates that to humiliate is "to lower the pride or self respect of; cause a painful loss of dignity to; mortify." To humiliate is to inflict shame—usually on another but in certain instances on oneself. Humiliation tends to be a triadic affair, requiring one who humiliates, one who is humiliated, and one witness (or more) whose good opinion is important to the one humiliated. Although it is possible for all three of these roles to be taken by the self, that is, one can be the perpetrator, victim, and witness of one's own humiliation (as with certain masochistic characters), normally when individuals feel humiliated, the roles of perpetrator and witness are taken by others (perpetrator and witness may be the same person or different persons). Morrison (1989) says that the one who humiliates must be important to the self; this may be so but need not be. It is sufficient that the good opinion of the witness to one's humiliation be important to the self—even if the self is the only witness. In some cases the one who humiliates may be a stranger or someone hated. Because humiliation tends to be a triadic affair, it is apt to be readily elicited in connection with the vicissitudes

75

of the oedipal situation, where it may play a role as important as, or more important than, castration anxiety in instigating various defensive operations.

The entire oedipal arena, the playground of classical psychoanalysis, is a mine field of potential shame and humiliation. The child, objectively speaking, is in the ridiculous position of having erotic ambitions that his or her size and immaturity render hopeless. Even were the child to emotionally triumph over his or her rival and be preferred by the coveted parent, shame is guaranteed by the child's inability to consummate the triumph. The ultimate repression or abandonment of the child's oedipal longing may have as much or more to do with shame/humiliation issues as with castration anxiety or guilt over hostile feelings toward the parent of the same gender.

Mayman (1975), in an unpublished paper, observed that for the male child at the phallic–oedipal stage shame experience is apt to center on a sense of the ludicrous insufficiency and the pathetic, childishly undeveloped state of the genitals, which the child might like to flaunt provocatively but fears others will find amusing or ridiculous.

Robert Stoller (1987) observed that

> Analytic theorists use "castration anxiety" as the dynamic that underlies the defenses of erotic life. Though it seems a most precise term, one that is evocative and full of drama, I find it lacks needed connotations. It points to anatomy when the issue is identity: who am I and is my "I" (selfhood) at risk? In muffling the identity meanings, "castration anxiety" fails to alert us to the shame/humiliation experiences that are the real essence of the sensed threats and the resulting reparative revenge fantasies. (p. 304)

Although I think Stoller is correct in calling needed attention to the shame/humiliation component in the dynamics of the oedipal situation, I would not like to go so far as to deny that castration anxiety is a real phenomenon in its own right or suggest that it can be entirely reduced to matters of shame/humiliation. I would prefer to say that the issue is anatomy *and* identity, their interrelationship. It is also important to recognize that shame may at times be used as a defense against castration

anxiety (Morrison, 1989) or even as a manifestation of castration anxiety.

HUMILIATION AND CHRISTIANITY

I believe that we cannot thoroughly understand the deeper significance of shame and humiliation in our culture without pay-
ing some attention to the influence of Christianity on the collective Western psyche. For example, Hillman (1983), pointing to
the repression of sexuality in the history of the Church, says
"Imagine a culture whose main God-image has no genitals and
whose Mother is sexually immaculate, Whose Father did not
sleep with his Mother" (p. 75). This, says Hillman is a collective
image that informs our cultural viewpoints and leaves a psychological heritage that we must deal with.

It is also instructive to meditate on aspects of the Passion
and Resurrection in our efforts to understand their collective
psychological residue. As a child I dreaded the weekly Lenten
services in which the ritual of the Stations of the Cross was
observed. Each station represented some scene from the Passion
and death of Christ. Bad enough that each station singled out
and celebrated some new physical or psychological suffering
inflicted on the Savior, but the celebration of all that humiliation
in addition to the suffering was too much for my young psyche.
Worse yet, one was exhorted to identify with this suffering,
murdered, and humiliated figure and to emulate him. And what
horrendous humiliation! Here was Christ, betrayed by those
close to him, spat upon, ridiculed, given a crown of thorns to
mock what his persecutors saw as his kingly pretensions, then
stripped and in his nakedness raised high on the cross, and
exposed to the gaze of all in his agony and death, while a carnival
atmosphere prevailed around him.

How could one be induced to identify with such a humiliated figure if it were not for the glory of the resurrected Christ?
In the Christian view Christ's suffering redeems mankind but,
psychologically speaking, it is also true that the glory of the
resurrected Christ redeems the image of the humiliated Christ.
Ignominious exposure and humiliation are expunged by glorious

77

exhibition to his disciples. Christ as teacher and miracle worker enjoyed considerable local fame prior to his humiliation, and that fame was highly relevant to the pleasure his tormentors took in mocking and humiliating him. The sequence of events was fame, followed by disgrace–humiliation, followed by glory.

In Christ we have a god image not only without functioning genitals, as Hillman notes, but a god-image laden with the core dynamic polarity of humiliation and death versus exhibited glory and eternal triumph. To the extent that Christian images tacitly shape the structure of our collective Western psyche, this image of the humiliated and glorious god has nuclear importance. This shame–glory complex is particularly observable in disorders of narcissism, as we shall see when we look at that issue in a later chapter. Understandably, most people prefer to emphasize the glorious aspect of the identification with the Christian god-image and reject the humiliation; at the deeper, unconscious level this is not so easily accomplished. The propensity of prominent Christian preachers and evangelists to bring disgrace and humiliation upon themselves (usually in connection with some sexual escapade) testifies to the power of this complex.

This theme of fame and exalted status followed by humiliation, followed by personal redemption through that humiliation can be found in Tom Wolfe's recent (1987) novel *The Bonfire of the Vanities*. In a powerfully drawn scene, Sherman McCoy, the protagonist of the novel, a successful, affluent, narcissistic Wall Street bond broker and self-proclaimed "master of the universe," is taken to the Bronx municipal building to be booked on a hit-and-run charge. There, handcuffed, standing in the pouring rain with drenched clothing, and waiting to be booked, he is tormented, abused, and mocked by reporters and photographers. His mortification is complete. McCoy's abject state is in sharp contrast to his earlier exalted status as "master of the universe" and one of New York's elite. After the psychic death (mortification) of the old Sherman McCoy and the destruction of his former life, we begin to see glimpses of a new resurrected Sherman McCoy—a more sympathetic figure, gutsier, more radical, perhaps happier. Whether Wolfe consciously intended it or not, his novel echoes an archetypally Christian theme.

· 7 ·

Shame, Psychoanalysis, and Psychotherapy

SHAME AND THE PSYCHOTHERAPY
OF NEUROTIC CHARACTER

Shapiro, in his most recent work (1989) on the psychotherapy of neurotic character, makes the point that it is the failure of the patient to adequately articulate the affective dimensions of his subjective experience that is involved in the maintenance of his neurosis. The clinical examples that Shapiro offers are nearly all instances in which the patient fails to articulate the experience of shame. In support of this claim let me offer this extended passage from Shapiro:

> What is needed, [to adequately understand neurosis] is a dynamic understanding, no longer of the dynamics of particular drive and defense but of the working of the personality as a whole. More specifically, the clinical facts seem to point to a neurotic self-estrangement of a different sort from the kind that is usually imagined. It is not an estrangement of a rational adult consciousness from an intrusive, now irrational childhood wish. It is a self-estrangement of a more general kind. It is a distortion or loss of self-awareness, an estrangement of reflective or articulated consciousness from the actuality of a largely unarticulated and diffuse subjective world. To put it more simply, it is an estrangement between what one *thinks* he feels or believes and what he *actually* feels or believes.

79

A middle-aged man of extremely sensitive pride is re-buffed by his boss. He declares himself to be—he thinks he is—"furious." But he looks far more humiliated and hurt than angry. This unarticulated and diffuse feeling of humilia-tion is not unconscious, strictly speaking. It is his actual subjective experience. Yet it is unrecognized by him. His pride prevents him from recognizing ("admitting," as he later says) the sensation of humiliation.

A woman, similarly sensitive, is much concerned about her comparatively low professional status and about being "pushed around" by others. She often speaks of herself as a "nobody." She is sincere when she describes herself that way. She is expressing what she thinks she believes, what in fact she often tells herself. But she does not believe it. She does not realize that in fact she constantly disparages her superiors and is contemptuous of them.

Another man constantly and anxiously measures and assures himself of his manliness. He has no awareness at all of the existence of that concern, however. His concern about his manliness continually, but without his notice, prompts him to reassure himself with thoughts about and actions to demonstrate his strong will and his accomplishments. This quasi-reflective process protects him from awareness of his concern.

These are all instances of self estrangement, instances in which the individual is cut off from himself. But in each case the estrangement is between the conscious idea of the self, of what one feels, on the one hand, and the actuality of subjec-tive experience, on the other. These are, again, distortions of self awareness. And they are produced by the internal dy-namics of the neurotic personality. (pp. 28–29)

In all three of the cases that Shapiro cites (and in nearly every clinical vignette in his book) the "internal dynamics" have to do with unacknowledged or unrecognized shame issues, what Lewis (1971) labeled bypassed shame; it is this which accounts for the self-estrangement that Shapiro describes as central to the neurotic process. As we have seen earlier, secondary shame about shame itself means that shame is apt to be the most unrecognized and unacknowledged of all the affects. Bypassed shame can be understood in terms of the operation of the defense mechanism of isolation, wherein the individual is caught up in obsessive ideation about the self but is not in touch with the affect driving that ideation. It is not just that we try to hide our shame from others but that we hide it from ourselves; or if we do recognize our shame experience, we fail to recognize the concomitant inflated estimate of our importance by which we compensate for that shame, as in the case of the woman cited earlier.

Although isolation of affect is one of the most frequent defense mechanisms employed in connection with shame, any defense mechanism may be used to protect oneself from shame experience. In the case of reaction formation we see "counter-shame" behavior, in which exaggerated pride, boastfulness, cultivated vulgarity, and exhibitionistic behavior replace denied shame. Projection and projective identification are also frequently called upon by some in dealing with shame, as we saw in Chapter 5.

Most recent books on working with shame in the clinical setting tend to focus on the patient's shame as a problem the patient brings with him when he enters the treatment setting and tend to neglect the interpersonal sources of shame in the therapeutic encounter itself. The problem of bypassed shame is not only a problem for patients but for therapists as well.

SOME GENERAL CONSIDERATIONS ABOUT SHAME IN THE TREATMENT SITUATION

In psychotherapy or psychoanalysis most patients experience significant tension and conflict that are created by the explicit or tacit demand for self-revelation and the threat of shame attending such revelation. Whether or not shame is elicited by self-exposure often depends more on the context of that exposure and the nature of the relationship with the person (or persons) before whom one is exposed than on the content of what is exposed. Whether the content of what is exposed is or is not shameful in the eyes of the patient, the response of the other (or absence of response), rather than the content of what is revealed is most often the primary source of shame.

In psychoanalysis and psychotherapy one often finds oneself unwittingly revealing more than one feels prepared to reveal;

this is a potential source of shame, since this exposure is not only an exposure to another but often a kind of self-revelation as well—one not necessarily welcomed. Schneider (1977), in the course of his extensive discussion of Freud's shameless handling of the famous Dora case, noted at one point that

> psychoanalysis is a system of interpretation that endeavors to uncover more about the individual than the individual knowingly and willingly chooses to disclose. It traffics in matters—dreams, slips of the tongue, symbolic gestures— which hint at more than the individual is consciously aware of. If one feels vulnerable to the psychoanalytic eye and ear, it is for good reason: one is constantly being led into further disclosure than one has chosen or consented to. (p. 102)

There is an ethical question involved, says Schneider, in thus being led into such unwilling disclosure. This was particularly true in Dora's case, since she was in therapy not because she wanted to be there but because, as Freud acknowledged, she was sent by her father and agreed to submit to analysis only out of respect for her father's authority.

Kramer (1990), who writes a monthly column for *The Psychiatric Times*, talked about his recent encounter with a child psychoanalyst his parent sent him to see when he was 12. Kramer seemed to recall little about that therapy; he did remember that he wanted to talk baseball, but his analyst insisted on talking about sex. While acknowledging that he derived some benefit from the therapy, Kramer (1990) had other reactions as well:

> There was, however, a coercive element to the therapy. I do not believe the coercion resided in any particular person. The expectation that I would share private thoughts with a stranger was coercive just because I was the kind of child who was likely to try to comply. Although the therapy helped me, I was angry and humiliated over it. Some of the forgetting may have begun there. (p. 5)

The situation in which one person addresses or attends to another opens the possibility of shame for both parties. As Tinder (1980) observed,

Through an act of address, one implies that the person addressed is not merely an object of experience and appraisal. But one whose address is rejected finds suddenly that he himself is such an object. Being ignored rather than actively rejected, is a variation on this experience, for one of the main characteristics of a mere object, as distinguished from a person, is that it may legitimately be left aside and accorded no attention.

An act of address, then, necessarily means running a risk. It may seem that an offer of attention is far safer, for a state of attention is comparatively passive and inconspicuous. This is perhaps true. Yet the difficulties of communication would be obscured were all risks assumed to lie on the side of address and none on the side of attention. An effective offer of attention has to be expressed, if only by a smile or a frown. For this to occur, the attention must be genuine; if it is merely affected, serious communication is apt to expose it as such. But a state of genuine attention is not easily attained. It requires interest and understanding; and hardest of all it requires humility, because without humility one cannot sincerely listen. All of these must be expressed, and there are multiple opportunities for failure. Hence to be addressed is to be an object of certain expectations and thus to suffer a kind of exposure. A failure to respond can bring a feeling of shame not unlike that to which one is vulnerable in an act of address. (pp. 153–154)

The relationship between therapist and patient is an asymmetrical one. The participants are unequal in many respects. By virtue of being in the practitioner's office the patient is admitting to suffering a degree of pain, distress, dysfunction, or dissatisfaction with himself that he has not been able to remedy by his own efforts at self-help. Such an admission is almost always the occasion of significant shame, whether acknowledged or not. The therapist, by contrast, is presumed to "have it all together" and to be more free of symptoms and problems than his patient. That this is often not the case in reality does not change the fact that these assumptions are imbedded in the psychotherapeutic set-up and are encouraged or promoted by that setup. The therapist/analyst is assumed to be the healthy one, the one who knows, the one who is objective, and the one who can show the patient the way out of his difficulties. The sense of inequality is further grounded in the therapist's possession of formal training and professional credentials, which the patient may lack.

Racker (1968) points out that rather than being an interaction between a sick person and a healthy one, analysis (and psychotherapy) is

> an interaction between two personalities, in both of which the ego is under pressure from the id, the superego, and the external world; each personality has its internal and external dependencies, anxieties and pathological defenses; each is also a child with its internal parents; and each of these whole personalities—that of the analysand and that of the analyst—responds to every event of the analytic situation. (p. 180)

Although Racker correctly points out the parity existing between patient and therapist, he sees as an essential difference the therapist's alleged "objectivity." Racker maintains that "true objectivity is based upon a form of internal division that enables the analyst to make himself (his own countertransference and subjectivity) the object of his continuous observation and analysis" (p. 180). The problem with this assertion is that it assumes that some kind of objective, neutral, observing part of the self or ego, *uncontaminated by the aforementioned subjectivity and countertransference,* can be split off from the rest of the personality at will. This argument simply begs the question of objectivity by assuming what it set out to prove, namely, that it is possible for the analyst to be objective about his patient because he can be objective about his own subjectivity. It is important to understand that the therapist's alleged objectivity is a myth. What actually obtains in the therapeutic situation is not objectivity but intersubjectivity.

If he is to benefit from the process, the patient is expected to reveal much about himself in the course of the therapy. There is no similar expectation about therapist self-disclosure, and most therapists (especially those of a psychoanalytic orientation) have been trained to refrain from deliberate or gratuitous self-disclosure. The rationale for curbing or severely limiting avoidable self-disclosure is based on the belief that the greater the amount of information available to the patient about the therapist's actual self, life situation, value system, and so forth, the less useful the therapist is as a transference object. According to this line of reasoning, the therapist must remain relatively anonymous in his personhood so that the patient may freely fantasize about him and project upon him whatever the patient needs to project in order to more clearly bring to light the patient's characteristic and unconsciously determined ways of perceiving others, which are based on earlier relationships with parental figures and other significant persons in the patient's early life. In other words, the less reality data the patient has to guide him in his perception of the therapist, the more the habitual unconscious biases (drives, wishes, defenses) influencing his perceptions of others and his behavior with them will be highlighted. A related rationale for severely limiting self-disclosure by the thrapist is that the more the patient knows about the therapist, his real-life situation, his values, interests, and so forth, the more the patient will, consciously or unconsciously, shape his communications to the therapist in accord with that knowledge, either to please and ingratiate or offend and defy. However valid this rationale for therapist anonymity may seem, this arrangement is shame inducing in both parties, although the shame of it often goes unrecognized or unacknowledged by both therapist and patient.

We might better understand how it is that the therapist's avoidance of self-exposure is an avoidance of shame experience and at the same time a source of shame if we take a brief historical excursion into the early days of psychoanalysis and appreciate the tensions leading to the formulation of the concept ot transference—as well as to the psychoanalytic arrangement of having the patient lie on a couch. Freud candidly admitted that the practice of having the patient lie on the couch rather than sit face-to-face with him sprang from his personal intolerance of being looked at by his patients all day long. As we know, the affect of shame is characterized by painful self-consciousness in which there is a strong wish to hide the face from the gaze of the other. Having the patient lie on the couch with the analyst sitting behind him is an arrangement that permits both parties to minimize their experience of the affect of shame. This arrangement is not without its problems, however.

85

On the one hand, by minimizing the patient's shame, the couch facilitates free association and better enables the patient to follow the basic rule of psychoanalysis, which is that the patient report whatever comes into his mind regardless of whether he considers it irrelevant, repugnant, or embarrassing (i.e., shame-inducing). On the other hand, the use of the couch mitigates or bypasses the affect of shame. The problem created by the use of the couch is that in bypassing shame one also bypasses the analysis of shame. I believe that Freud's sensitivity to shame, which resulted in the physical arrangement of the patient on the couch and analyst safely out of view, led him to collude with the patient in the avoidance of shame analysis.

SHAME AND THE TRANSFERENCE

The concept of transference emerged historically from Freud's need to find a way of managing the troublesome situation in which the analyst became the focus of the patient's highly charged erotic interests. As the informed student of psychoanalytic history knows, Freud's collaborator in the early development of psychoanalysis, Joseph Breuer, reportedly broke off his relationship with his famous patient "Anna O" in response to his wife's increasing displeasure over his lively interest in his engaging young patient. According to Jones (1953), after informing Anna O of his intention to end the treatment, Breuer was summoned back to her house later the same day to find her in the throes of hysterical childbirth, the outcome of a pregnancy fantasy that had been silently developing in the context of her relationship with Breuer. Breuer allegedly fled the scene in a cold sweat and the following day (according to Jones) took his wife to Venice for a second honeymoon.

Jones (1953) further reveals that

> Confirmation of this account may be found in a contemporary letter Freud wrote to Martha, which contains substantially the same story. She at once identified herself with Breuer's wife, and hoped the same thing would not ever happen to her, whereupon Freud reproved her

vanity in supposing other women would fall in love with
her husband: for that to happen one has to be a Breuer.
(p. 225)

Many years later, in attempting to persuade Breuer to give
to the world the discovery Breuer and his patient Anna O had
made concerning the cathartic method, Freud encountered
strong resistance on Breuer's part, which Freud gradually recognized as having to do with Breuer's disturbing experience with
Anna O. Freud overcame Breuer's reservations by telling of his
own experience of a female patient passionately flinging her arms
around his neck in an impulsive moment (Freud had obviously
learned in the meantime that one doesn't have to be a Breuer for
that to happen) and explained to Breuer his reasons for regarding
such happenings as transference phenomena. According to Jones
(1953), Breuer's introduction to the concept of transference had
a calming effect on him, since he "evidently had taken his own
experience of the kind more personally and perhaps even re-
proached himself for indiscretion in the handling of his patient"
(p. 250).

Rather than require either patient or analyst to break off the
relationship to avoid the feeling of engaging in some kind of
illicit, unprofessional, or immoral kind of interaction (which
might possibly lead to explicit sexual intimacy or require that the
analyst directly reject the patient's interest and thus wound or
humiliate the patient), the concept of transference enabled the
analyst to remain on the scene as analyst while fleeing the scene
as person.

Szasz (1963) observed that

in psychoanalysis what stands between obscenity and science
is the concept of transference. This concept and all it implies, renders the physician a nonparticipant with the patient
in the latter's preoccupation with primary emotions (such as
eroticism, aggression, etc.). Only by not responding to the
patient on his own level of discourse and instead analyzing
his productions does the analyst raise his relationship with
the patient to a higher level of experience. . . . The concept
of transference was reassuring for another reason as well. It
introduced into medicine and psychology the notion of the

87

therapist as symbol; this renders the therapist as person
essentially invulnerable. (p. 35)

It is difficult to escape the conclusion that if transference hadn't
been "discovered," it would have to have been invented. By interpreting the patient's love and desire for him, or antagonism and
animosity, as transference, the therapist not only renders himself,
as person, invulnerable but also rationalizes the distancing and
rejection inherent in his refusal to discourse on the same level as
the patient. The therapist says, in effect, "I am not personally
rejecting you by failing to accept or respond to your feelings on a
more personal level, because your feelings are not really meant for
me (personally) at all but are merely revived feelings for earlier
figures in your life; I only serve as symbol of those earlier figures
by virtue of your projection onto me of characteristics of those
persons." This is almost invariably experienced (at some level) by
the patient as a devious, indirect rejection on the part of the therapist that evokes as intense (or even more intense) a feeling of shame
and humiliation as would attend a more direct rejection. The only
difference is that the transference interpretation makes it likely
that the shame and humiliation that may be evoked by the interpretation will be effectively denied, since the transference interpretation implicitly denies that any "real" rejection is taking place.
    Unacknowledged shame and humiliation lead to unarticu-
lated rage, the source of which may be only dimly grasped by the
patient, and this rage toward the therapist is apt to be guilt-
producing because it is experienced by the patient as irrational
and unjustified. This sequence of shame/humiliation, followed
by rage, followed by guilt has been well described and illustrated
by Lewis (1971). Negative therapeutic reaction is the term used to
refer to the situation in which the patient apparently gets worse
as the result of what the analyst considers valid and well-timed
interpretations. I believe that much of what is designated as
negative therapeutic reaction has its source in the unrecognized
shame dynamics I have been discussing.
    In his book on psychoanalytic technique, Greenson (1967),
offered the following illustration of the "compassionate firm-
ness" required of the analyst in his approach to the positive
transference. It is instructive on many levels.

88

A young woman, shy and timid, begins in the third month of her analysis to evince unmistakable signs of believing that she has fallen in love with me. Finally, after some days of struggling with her feelings, she tearfully confesses her love. Then she begs me not to treat this state of affairs in the same cold analytic way I had treated her other emotions. *She pleads with me not to remain silent and aloof.* I should please say something, anything—*it is so humiliating for her to be in such a position.* She weeps and sobs and becomes silent. *After a while* I say "I know this is very hard for you, but it is important for us that you try to express exactly how you feel." The patient is silent a moment and then says pleadingly and angrily: "It's not fair, you can hide behind the analytic couch and I have to expose all. I know you don't love me but at least tell me if you like me; admit you care a little, tell me I'm not just a number to you—the eleven o'clock patient." She weeps and sobs and is silent again. *I too keep silent for a time* and then say: "It's true it is not fair; the analytic situation is not an equal one: it is your task to let your feelings come out and it is my job to understand you, to analyze what comes up. Yes, It's not fair."

This remark of mine seemed to help the patient. She could then express more of her anger and sense of outrage. *The succeeding hours had mixtures of love and hate in them* but she became able to work on these reactions. . . . After I admitted to her that the analytic situation was not fair in the sense that she had to expose herself and I had the job of analyzing her, she tried to resume expressing her feelings of love for me. *But now a note of anger was added to her sad, pleading, urgent tone; I could hear an undertone of bitterness:* "I know you are right, I should let myself go, no matter how you feel about it. *It is so hard to cry out for love, to beg, and only to get silence as a response.* But after all you must be used to this, I suppose this happens with all your patients. I wonder how you can stand it . . . but after all you get paid for listening." (pp. 226–227; emphasis mine)

Although Greenson, to his credit, acknowledges the "unfairness" of the analytic situation he fails to really address with his patient the nature of that unfairness, that is, that it inflicts shame and humiliation on the patient while protecting the analyst from the risks of similar exposure. Greenson does not really address his patient's humiliation in any direct way although he is not unaware of the humiliating aspects of the analytic situation.

He candidly admits at one point in his book that "the analytic procedure is inevitably a one-sided, demeaning experience for the patient" (p. 278). Greenson's patient, at the moment of her greatest shame and vulnerability, begs him not to remain silent and aloof; he nevertheless responds to her pleas with silence, presumably not to provide her with a transference gratification. "One cannot permit even the most innocent and partial of erotic gratifications" (p. 226), says Greenson, citing Freud's recommendations. By leaving her in silence at the moment when she is feeling most vulnerable to humiliation the analyst delivers the humiliation she dreads. As we saw earlier, receiving no response from the other whom one is addressing is a form of rejection; it is characteristic of an object that it can be ignored, and shame, as we have emphasized, is intimately connected with the sense of being objectified or depersonified. Greenson notes the subsequent appearance of hate, anger, and resentment in the patient's communications—a clear response to the humiliation inflicted on her in the name of analysis. This vignette clearly illustrates that the so-called negative transference is often not transference at all, in the sense of an inappropriate displacement onto the person of the analyst of negative feelings properly belonging to earlier figures in the patient's life, but is instead a response to the shame and humiliation perpetrated on the patient by the analyst by means of his analytic technique. The patient's present humiliation in the treatment setting will usually evoke many painful memories of earlier humiliations, but one is not entitled to infer from this that the patient's shame response to the behavior of the analyst is primarily a transference phenomenon. Greenson (1967) seems to do exactly that in the following vignette:

> A young man, Mr. Z, reports he is annoyed at me for charging him for a missed hour. I pursue this "annoyance," questioning him if he really means annoyed. He "guesses" he was more than annoyed. My silence prods him into expressing rather heatedly how he thought I am a hypocrite for pretending to be a scientist. I am just as much a businessman as his "tight-assed" old man. Someday he hopes he'll have the courage to rub my nose in all this "psychoanalytic crap." This would be a fine revenge, he would do to me what I am doing to him. To my question: "And what am I doing to

you?'' he answers: "You make me crawl through all the shit, you never let up, more, more, more. You're never satisfied, produce or get out is what you seem to be saying and it's never enough." One can see behind the innocent annoyance he "guesses" he had the anal-sadistic fury and humiliation of childhood.

This same patient, later on in his analysis, begins his hour by stating he hated to come, he hates the analysis and me along with it. When I ask him: "And how do you hate me today?" he answers Today he hates me with a passion, a cold rage. He wouldn't want to kill me, no that would be too civilized. He would like to beat me to a pulp, literally grind me up into a jelly like a mass of bloody, slimy "goo." Then he'd eat me in one big "slurp" like the goddamned oatmeal his mother made him eat as a kid. Then he'd shit me out as a foul-smelling poisonous shit. And when I ask him: "And what would you do with this foul-smelling, poisonous shit?" he replied: "I'd grind you into the dirt so you could join my dear dead mother!" (p. 304)

Is this patient's perception of the analysis as so overwhelmingly humiliating and the cold rage he feels about that humiliation simply a transference phenomenon? We can not comfortably draw such a conclusion, because of the fact that the traditional psychoanalytic setup inflicts considerable shame and humiliation on the patient. By Greenson's own admission the analytic procedure is an inevitably demeaning experience for the patient.

Consider the following two vignettes, which Greenson offers as examples of "clarification of the transference."

A patient tells me she had a thought of "kissing" my "genital organ." At the appropriate moment I asked her to please explain what she meant by kissing my penis, I found her statement vague and somewhat evasive. I indicate by my question that I want to know the intimate details and that it is permissible to talk of them in a realistic way. I demonstrate this by the way I talk. I am neither vulgar nor evasive. I help her on her way by translating "genital organ" into "penis." The "kissing" she will have to translate herself.

A male patient tells me he had a "fellatio" fantasy about me. When I feel it is indicated I tell him I do not understand what he means by "fellatio," would he please explain this to me. When he hems and haws, I say that he seems to have difficulty talking about doing something sexual with his mouth to my penis. By so doing, I not only point out his transference resistance but also indicate how I would like him to be able to talk of such matters in concrete, everyday, living language. (p. 303)

Is this "clarification of the transference" or rationalized humiliation? Greenson would surely deny that his intention in this instance was to humiliate the patient; nevertheless, he does not follow the usual analytic principal of analyzing defense before content, which would require that he deal with the patient's shame and embarrassment before worrying about the specific details of the patient's sexual fantasy. This is reflective of the insufficient attention shame has traditionally received in psychoanalysis.

Szasz (1963) made the point that the concept of transference harbors the seeds of its own destruction and of the destruction of psychoanalysis itself. This is so, says Szasz, because it tends to place the person of the analyst beyond the reality testing of his patient. The analyst attempts to claim the right of being pure subject and to thus escape the possible shame of objectification. The analytic setup operates on the assumption that the patient's perceptions and assessments of the analyst are badly skewed by virtue of the transference whereas the analyst's perceptions of the patient and himself are, for the most part, veridical. The patient is objectified but the analyst seeks, by means of the concept of transference, to spare himself similar objectification and the shame that might accompany such objectification.

Simply put, whatever other value it might have (and undeniably it does have other value), the concept of transference has to be looked at as a defense against shame, and that is why it has been so "idealized" by psychoanalysis and why it became the cornerstone of psychoanalytic treatment. "It is impossible to destroy anyone in absentia or in effigie," said Freud (1912, p. 108). By that he meant that transference phenomena make "the patient's hidden and forgotten erotic impulses immediate and manifest," and thereby bring the neurosis into the present moment where it can be more effectively confronted and resolved. However, the same statement "It is impossible to destroy anyone in absentia or in effigie," could also be understood on another level as a statement about the defensive function of transference for the analyst. The concept of transference enables the analyst to absent himself as person from the situation and substitute in his stead an effigy of the patient's old libidinal objects, thus protecting himself from feeling personally engaged (destroyed?) by the patient's erotic or aggressive inclinations. He also thereby protects himself from the destructive power of the shame he might experience were he to allow himself to be drawn into a discourse on the same level as the patient.

Because the concept of transference is in the public domain and familiar to most educated people, many patients try to protect themselves from the possible shame and sense of rejection implicit in transference interpretations by identification with the aggressor: They immediately interpret any strong feelings toward the therapist as transference manifestations, beating the therapist to the interpretation they fear and thus protecting themselves. The following exchange illustrates this self-protective response.

SARAH: I think I'm developing transference feelings for you.

FB: What do you mean?

SARAH: You know what I mean. Transference.

FB: Transference . . . isn't that what you use to get from one bus to another?

SARAH: (*laughs*) You know what I mean. Your female patients are supposed to fall in love with you. It's supposed to happen to everybody in therapy. You must see it all the time.

FB: By talking about what *everybody* feels you seem to be avoiding talking about *your* feelings.

SARAH: I feel so stupid. I know this is supposed to happen to everybody, but I don't like it happening to me. I don't want to be just like all your other patients. You probably find it amusing.

FB: You still seem to be avoiding being more specific about your feelings. Your reference to feeling stupid suggests that you're feeling embarrassed. You're apparently afraid that I'll laugh at your feelings.

SARAH: Well, I am very attracted to you and I find myself thinking about you a great deal of the time. I know this happens when people go into therapy but you must think "Ho hum, here we go again."

FB: You seem to believe that I will fail to respond to you as an individual but only as an example of some textbook phenomenon.

SARAH: Exactly. I'm afraid that you're going to tell me that my feelings are really for my father or something like that. (*laughs*)

FB: I would be too embarrassed to make such a trite statement.

In the normal course of developing intimacy between two persons there is a reciprocal process of self-disclosure, roughly based on a quid pro quo rule. If A expresses feeling, desires, and fantasies about B and B fails to respond at a similar level, then A is apt to feel shame. At some level of his being, B is also apt to feel unacknowledged shame for failing to meet A on the same level of discourse and self-disclosure.

Tomkins (1963), enumerated the sources of shame arising from love, friendship, and close interpersonal relationships:

> If I wish to touch you but you do not wish to be touched, I may feel ashamed. If I wish to look at you but you do not wish me to, I may feel ashamed. If I wish you to look at me but you do not, I may feel ashamed. If I wish to look at you and at the same time wish that you look at me, I can be shamed. If I wish to be close to you but you move away, I am ashamed. If I wish to suck or bite your body and you are reluctant, I can become ashamed. If I wish to hug you or you hug me or we hug each other and you do not reciprocate my wishes, I feel ashamed. If I wish to have sexual intercourse with you but you do not, I am ashamed.
>
> If I wish to hear your voice but you will not speak to

me, I can feel shame. If I wish to speak to you but you will not listen, I am ashamed. If I would like us to have a conversation but you do not wish to converse, I can be shamed. If I would like to share my ideas, aspirations or my values with you but you do not reciprocate, I am ashamed. If I wish to talk and you wish to talk at the same time, I can become ashamed. If I want to tell you my ideas but you wish to tell me yours, I can become ashamed.

If I want to share my experiences with you but you wish to tell me your philosophy of life, I can become ashamed. If I wish to speak of personal feelings but you wish to speak about science, I will feel ashamed. If you wish to talk about the past and I wish to dream about the future, I can become ashamed. (p. 192)

The variety of shame sources in interpersonal interaction that Tomkins identifies gives us a better sense of how the frustration of devoutly sought mutuality, reciprocity, or complementarity can evoke shame. By refusing to join his patient on the same level of discourse the therapist is guaranteeing that his patient will not lack for abundant shame experiences. If the shame experiences evoked by the asymmetrical and hierarchical nature of the therapeutic relationship were made thematic for the therapy, the therapeutic gain realized from the analysis of these shame dynamics would seem to justify and honor the shame suffered by the patient. Unfortunately, this doesn't happen very often.

In addition to the shame of unrequited interest, desire, and intimate disclosure, there is another dynamic force that underlies the patient's resistance to the erotic "transference." I am referring to the self's struggle against surrendering to the power of archetypal insistancies, which are feared as bringing about an unacceptable loss of control, the result of an internal revolution in which the ego is dethroned and delivered over to the irresistible enthrallment with the other. This is characteristically experienced as a shameful loss of freedom, an entrapment, enslavement, or imprisonment. It is the ego's shame and humiliation in the face of this lack of control, finding itself in the grip of an impersonal force more powerful than itself, that constitutes one of the principle resistances to the development and acknowledgment of the erotic transference.

SOURCES OF SHAME
FOR THE ANALYST/THERAPIST
IN THE TREATMENT SITUATION

Does the therapist invariably experience shame (acknowledged or unacknowledged) for failing to meet his patient on the same level of discourse and self-disclosure? I believe that at some level of his being this is likely to be the case; his shame may be well articulated, marginally conscious, or largely unconscious. Occasionally, it surfaces in the form of some uncharacteristic burst of self-disclosure. The therapist's shame is activated by his nagging realization that by shunning self-disclosure, by not sharing "countertransference," and by interpreting the patient's interests and emotional experiences with him as transference phenomena, he, the therapist, is "hiding" and attempting to render himself as a person invulnerable. He is refusing to be an object and insisting on being a subject only. This sought-after invulnerability is both invulnerability to shame and invulnerability to the temptation to use the patient for gratification of personal need or desire, which would also be shame- and guilt-generating. The more strongly the therapist must defend against the shame he feels for his avoidance of self-disclosure and the guilt he feels for inflicting shame on the patient, the more strongly he is apt to idealize the transference and what is sometimes refered to as "the frame," that is, the ground rules that include therapist anonymity, confidentiality, neutrality, strict time and payment arrangements, and so forth.

The therapist is caught in the paradoxical situation where the failure to join the patient at the same level of discourse is apt to be shame-inducing but to do so might also be shame- and guilt-inducing. The therapist must recognize this paradox and learn to live with it without trying to eliminate it. Too rigid efforts to avoid self-disclosure of any kind reflect the therapist's exaggerated search for invulnerability and his desire to be subject alone whereas too liberal and undisciplined self-disclosure is more apt to be in the service of the therapist's need for affirmation and understanding and may well be seductive in nature.

The therapist is also vulnerable to shame to the extent that he cannot offer significant help to his patient; he has to confront the limitations of his knowledge and techniques—and, possibly, also those unresolved personal problems that interfere with his ability to assist the patient. He is vulnerable to shame not only with regard to the limitations of his personal knowledge and skill; as he gains more experience, he may begin to entertain disquieting doubts about the knowledge and skill of his teachers and his own analyst and about the state of the art in general. It is something of a professional crisis, to say the least, when one realizes that a great deal of what one was taught concerning the way to conduct therapy or analysis really doesn't work and that the received theory with which one has operated is quite inadequate. A de-idealization of one's former role models and professional heroes often takes place as part of such a crisis, and de-idealization is frequently accompanied by a vague feeling of shame.

Janet Malcolm's (1980) book *Psychoanalysis: The Impossible Profession*, is based in large part on interviews with an anonymous New York analyst to whom she assigned the pseudonym of Aaron Green. Malcom writes:

> And yet apparently the work of analysis, for all its comfortable distance and non-involvement, is oddly unpleasant and agitating. Analysts are plagued by doubt and anxiety. "The gestalt of the profession is guilt," Aaron said. "Guilt over not understanding the patient. Analysts always suspect themselves of not being in control of the plethora of material coming out of the patient. They are being paid and trusted to perform a therapeutic service and they are in the dark about certain things about the patient. There may be a rattlesnake under that rock, and they don't see it. This kind of thing is devastating, and it's chronic. Everybody worries about it. It's talked about, in an extremely guarded way, whenever analysts get together in small groups. It is in these small groups that ambiguities and self-doubts come out. You don't hear about them at the meetings of the American Psychoanalytic Association or of the International. (p. 111)

Green here commits the error, one that is epidemic in psychoanalytic writing, of labeling as guilt what would be more accurately identified as shame. The analyst's chronic feelings of ignorance, confusion, and inadequacy that Green refers to are more rightly a source of shame rather than guilt. Once again guilt has swallowed up shame.

THE PROBLEM OF INTERPRETATION

A single professional woman in her early 30s has been in psychotherapy for about a year. In a recent hour she referred to a disturbing dream. She struggled for several minutes with head down and gaze averted before she could report to me the following dream.

> I am in the rest room in this building (where the therapist's office is located). I am trying to insert this amputated penis into my vagina but there is an obstruction which makes it difficult to accomplish. As I leave the rest room someone, a plainclothes policeman or detective, approaches me and says there is a rapist in the building and they want to use me as a decoy. While I'm waiting for the rapist to appear I'm still trying to insert this penis under my skirt, hoping nobody will notice the bulge in my crotch. This suspicious-looking macho character appears and he's following some woman so I assume this is the guy. I take off my blouse and approach him bare-breasted, saying seductively, "Look what I've got here." I start rubbing his chest and then his genitals, and I say to him, "They're rather small, aren't they?" He looks hurt and angry.

This patient rarely reports dreams and when she does offer a dream, she produces little or nothing in the way of associations. True to form, she offered no associations to this dream except to speculate that inserting the amputated penis into her vagina might represent a kind of abortive attempt at sexual intercourse of a sort. This patient has been leading a very celibate life for many years, with no romantic or sexual involvements. She works in a male-dominated professional world and her professional self is the only aspect of her person that she values. In the hours preceding this dream we had been discussing her rejection of her femaleness as reflected in her aversion to bonding to other females or identifying herself with female groups or female interests. As I listened to the patient's dream, I thought that the dream had to do with the issue of female castration, shame, humiliation, and defensive exhibitionism. I thought of the amputated penis as her own "lost" penis, the penis she imagined she once had, and her attempts to insert it in her vagina as an effort at restoration of what had been lost, an effort that was being obstructed by something (the therapy or therapist?). Her hope that nobody would notice the bulge in her crotch seemed to reflect the wish that neither I nor others would recognize her powerful male strivings and identifications (her hidden penis), or, at a deeper level, that no one would notice the absence of a penis, her shamefully defective state. All of this pointed to significant shame over perceived genital defectiveness in her early development, a theme Freud recognized and universalized when he called shame "a feminine characteristic par excellence." The seductive exhibition of her breasts seemed an effort to distract attention from her genitals. "Look at what I've got here" (breasts) seemed to imply "Don't look at what I haven't got down here (genitals)." In other words, it was a defensive act of exhibitionism motivated by shame and designed more to conceal than to reveal. The shame of genital deficiency was projected in the last part of the dream and the tables were turned; it was the macho male who was humiliated by her cutting comment, designed to make him feel genitally inadequate. I also suspected that the macho male rapist whom she wished to humiliate might represent me, since the dream took place in the building where my office is located. All of these thoughts were, of course, my own unspoken interpretations, based not on her associations to the dream, since she produced hardly any, but on my previous experience with the patient and my theoretical grounding in psychoanalytic theory. I asked myself, How much of this interpretation should I offer the patient?

I decided to approach the dream in this way: I said to her that this dream was about shame and humiliation. I pointed out that she announced this in advance by her visible shame reaction before telling me about the dream (lowered head, averted gaze, long delay, and so forth). I then slowly began to share with her most of my thoughts about her dream. She listened quietly and attentively, apparently reflecting on what I said. She neither disputed nor affirmed this line of interpretation but said something to the effect that she is amazed by how much can be gleaned from a dream. Sitting on the sofa, she slowly drew her legs up toward her chest and lowered her head to her knees, hiding her face. She remained silent and in response to my inquiry as to what was going on with her she mutely shook her head. I interpreted her posture and silence as withdrawal and concealment resulting from feeling overexposed by her dream and by my interpretation of the dream. This unexpected overexposure, I said, had elicited more shame. I suggested that it was her effort to avoid the kind of shame experience that she was now feeling that made her reluctant to bring dreams to her therapy hours, and to provide associative clues to the dreams she did bring. I added that I also suspected that it was my ability to understand the dream, when it was incomprehensible to her, that evoked in her a sense of inferiority that was a source of still further shame. She was such a passive nonparticipant during this part of the process that I felt, while I was making all these interpretations, that I was acting like a kind of psychic rapist— was that why I was so represented in the patient's dream? I felt uneasy about this but reminded myself that the patient in the throes of strong shame affect is basically "incommunicado," unable to effectively verbalize what is going on with him, and that the therapist must then verbalize what the patient is unable to. Still, I felt troubled and wondered if I was feeling like a psychic rapist out of identification with some projection of the patient or if I was feeling like one because I was indeed acting like one? I also began to suspect that her lack of response to my interpretations might be the equivalent of telling the rapist that his genitals were too small. Was my guilt over feeling like a rapist a cover for shame over feeling ineffectual?

The preceding vignette is an illustration of an interpretive process guided by attention to the affect of shame—the patient's shame to be sure, but the therapist's shame as well. It also illustrates some of the hazards of interpretation in general.

The act of interpretation involves the reformulation of a given psychic event, dream, symptom, personal statement, or action from its immediate subjective meaning for the patient to a more impersonal, objective, experience-distant, theoretical framework. The therapist interpreting in the light of his theoretical leanings is always involved to a degree in an objectification of the patient that is apt to be shame-inducing. To the extent that the therapist considers interpretation to be his primary task, he will need to be especially sensitive to shame dynamics. Kohutian self psychologists often tend to de-emphasize the importance of interpretation, particularly interpretation from an "objective" position outside the patient's perspective, in favor of empathic immersion in the material from within the patient's subjective perspective. Remaining empathically attuned to the patient's perspective is the essence of being a satisfactory "selfobject." Interpretation by definition brings an additional "outside" perspective to the situation and involves a reframing or reordering of the material of the session; hence, it may be experienced by the patient as a selfobject failure.

An understanding of the patient's reaction to interpretation may be more important than the validity of the interpretation itself. As I said earlier, an individual must, if he is to lead a fully responsible life, accept being both subject and object and thus confront what Lichtenstein (1963) called the dilemma of human identity. Many problems arise from the efforts of individuals to evade the living exchange of being both subject and object by trying to be either subject only or object only. Interpretation, since it involves an element of objectification, may be more negatively received by the person who insists on being subject only and insists that all situations must be seen exclusively from his perspective. On the other hand, the person who has elected to be object only will blindly and uncritically assume that outside perspectives are inherently more accurate than personal subjective ones and will docilely submit to the element of objectification inherent in interpretation.

The art of interpretation seems to me to involve the ability on the part of the therapist to convey to the patient that he, the therapist, understands the patient's subjective perspective and associated affect state while at the same time widening the frame of that perspective to include hitherto excluded considerations. To use the terminology introduced earlier, ideally the patient needs to experience himself as a SUBJECT–object to the therapist, rather than a subject–OBJECT or OBJECT only. Classical psychoanalytic theory is an objectifying theory that seeks to explain all human behavior in terms of universal drive–defense conflicts mediated by certain psychic structures. When one interprets from within the framework of classical psychoanalytic theory, the patient's struggles are interpreted as particular instantiations or exemplification of these universal drive–defense conflicts. The uniqueness of the patient's own subjective world may not receive adequate recognition or affirmation. What does not lend itself to interpretation within the framework of established psychoanalytic theory is apt to be simply ignored or passed over. The patient is likely to experience himself as a subject–OBJECT or OBJECT for the therapist or analyst who operates within this kind of framework, leading to shame and muted shame–rage.

Any theory that seeks to interpret an individual's actions by invoking universal explanatory principles is apt to evoke significant patient resistance when applied in the psychotherapy situation because of its built-in objectification. The nature of science is to establish universal explanatory principles, but the aim of the individual in psychotherapy is to be understood within the framework of his own subjectivity and individuality. The art of psychotherapy lies in the ability to satisfy this need of the patient to be a SUBJECT–object without having to sacrifice hard-won insights about human psychodynamics of a more universal nature.

·IV·

Psychoanalysis, Shame, and Society

·8·

Shame and Sexuality

SHAME AND ITS RELATIONSHIP TO
VOYEURISM AND EXHIBITIONISM

What about the idea that shame is a reaction formation against voyeurism and/or exhibitionism, which Freud put forward and subsequent analysts have echoed? Straus (1980), as I mentioned in Chapter 1, has contested the notion that voyeurism and exhibitionism are normal components of the sexual drive, and he has argued that they reflect an alteration in communicative mode, involving distancing and objectification. Straus writes that "The looking of the voyeur . . . is as different from the looks exchanged by lovers as medical palpation from a gentle caress of the hand. In [voyeuristic] viewing there is a transition from the immediate I–thou relationship to the subject–object relationship proper" (p. 219).

It is undoubtedly true that a healthy *sense of shame* defends against voyeuristic and exhibitionistic activities of various kinds, but it also seems to be true that strong and enduring *shame affect* may fuel voyeuristic and exhibitionistic activities.

Sex, Lies, and Videotapes is a recent film that offers significant insight into the relationship between voyeurism and sexual love. In the film we are introduced to four main characters. John, a scudsy young lawyer, is sexually involved with Cynthia, the promiscuous, cynical sister of his wife, Ann; Ann is a sympathetic, "wholesome," trusting type, somewhat shy and inhibited in sexual matters (by modern standards) but with a passionate nature; the fourth character, Graham, is an old college buddy of John's who drifts into town. It becomes immediately apparent that he and and John have little in common anymore, but he and Ann are drawn to one another. Graham confesses to Ann that he has been impotent for many years and does not even attempt sex with women anymore. Ann later discovers to her dismay and revulsion that his sexual gratification consists in masturbating while watching videotapes of women he has personally interviewed about their sex lives. These women not only discuss their sexual histories but sometimes volunteer to undress or masturbate on camera. Graham's impotence and the constriction of his sexuality to voyeurism, the film suggests, are related to an earlier love disappointment with a woman named Elizabeth, a disappointment perhaps based on some kind of betrayal.

The film wryly contrasts Ann's acceptance of her therapist's "professional" voyeurism when he quizzes her about her masturbatory activities with her initial rejection of Graham's more honest but kinky brand of voyeurism. Ann suspects that John is involved with her sister; but when she questions him, he lies to her and feigns indignation. When Ann later finds proof of his sexual relationship with her sister, she is outraged as much by his lying as by his infidelity. Her respect for Graham's honesty and her rage at her husband lead her to go to Graham and volunteer to be interviewed by him on videotape. The interview begins but soon roles are reversed, and Ann is interviewing Graham about his sexual difficulties. At one point as she quizzes him, she turns the camera on him, something he finds intolerably objectifying and maddening. Backed by a sense of trust and honesty, Ann moves closer to him to initiate sexual intimacy. At this point he discreetly turns off the camera.

Later, in a fit of rage following John's disclosure that he had "fucked" Graham's great lost love, Elizabeth, a woman who "knew how to keep a secret," Graham trashes his videotapes, an act symbolizing his freedom from the constricted sexuality of the voyeur and his newfound ability to engage Ann in a more integrated emotional and sexual relationship. The film clearly suggests that Graham's voyeurism was connected to his earlier betrayal at the hands of Elizabeth and that out of that injury to himself, resulting in a damaged sense of trust, he moved into the altered relational mode of the voyeur, objectifying women and distancing himself from them sexually while trying to discover their sexual secrets. Betrayal of trust and dishonesty served to rupture what Kaufman (1985) called *the interpersonal bridge,* resulting in the experience of shame. Instead of shame being a reaction formation to voyeurism, voyeurism in Graham's case was a reaction to shame.

Clinical experience teaches us that fear, shame, and lack of trust in the opposite gender seem to fuel voyeuristic and exhibitionistic perversions. I use the word *perversion* to refer to those cases in which looking or exhibiting is the primary, essential, or exclusive means of obtaining sexual satisfaction. Instead of shame being simply a reaction formation defending against voyeurism and exhibitionism, shame appears to be the driving affect leading to voyeuristic and exhibitionistic behavior, at least in the case of perversions. Freud seems to have gotten it backwards or, at best, only partly right.

A REAPPRAISAL OF THE RELATIONSHIP BETWEEN SHAME AND SEXUALITY

Because excessive shame about sexual matters may seriously interfere with a person's sexual functioning, shame has been simplistically viewed as the enemy of healthy sexuality. We are a long way from Freud's fin de siècle Vienna and the sexual mores and hypocrisies of that time; given our own very different problems with sexuality, perhaps it is time we reconsidered the relationship between shame and sexuality.

The most incisive critique of modern attitudes toward sexuality that I have read is to be found in Leslie Farber's (1976) mordantly witty and deliciously ironic essay "I'm Sorry Dear," which is essential reading for anyone who wants to understand what has happened to sex in our times. Farber writes:

> My conviction is that over the last fifty years sex has, for the most part, lost its viability as a human experience. I do not mean that there is any danger that it will cease to be practiced—that it will be put aside like other Victorian bric-a-

brac. The hunger will remain, perhaps even increase, and human beings will continue to couple with as much fervor as they can provoke, while the human possibilities of sex will grow ever more elusive. (p. 125)

In his analysis of where we went wrong Farber concluded that the industrial revolution of the 19th century, with its concern for the health and sickness of the machine, powered by steam and electricity, came more and more to view the human body as another machine. When it was decided that the dominant energy source of this machine was sexual, the science of sexology was born. Granting that it had always been medicine's privilege to regard the body as a natural object with many machine-like characteristics, Farber makes the following point:

> But, for the first time, scientists, in their intoxication, could forget the duality previous centuries knew: namely, that the body is and is not a natural object . . . With the suppression of the second half of the dialectic, sexology and psychoanalysis could—with the assistance of the romantics—claim the erotic life as their exclusive province, removing it from all the traditional disciplines, such as religion, philosophy, and literature, which had always concerned themselves with sex as human experience. *Such qualities as modesty, privacy, reticence, abstinence, chastity, fidelity, and shame could now be questioned as rather arbitrary matters that interfered with the health of the sexual parts.* (p. 141, emphasis mine)

Is the association between shame and sexuality only an arbitrary, learned relationship that we should have unlearned by now, in our more enlightened and sexually free age? Those whose thinking is thoroughly shaped by Freudian doctrine would undoubtedly answer in the affirmative. (Freud's basic views on shame were reviewed in earlier chapters.) In order to deepen our understanding of the issues concerning shame and sexuality, let us examine a passage from Freud's (1905/1953) "Three Essays on the Theory of Sexuality"

> It has been brought to our notice that we have been in the habit of regarding the connection between the sexual instinct and the sexual object as more intimate than it in fact is.

108

Experience of the cases that are considered abnormal has shown us that in them the sexual instinct and the sexual object are merely soldered together—a fact which we have been in danger of overlooking in consequence of the uniformity of the normal picture, where the object appears to form part and parcel of the instinct. *We are thus warned to loosen the bond that exists in our thought between instinct and object.* It seems probable that the sexual instinct is in the first instance independent of its object; nor is its origin likely to be due to its object's attractions. (pp. 147–148, emphasis mine)

In discussing this passage, Davidson (1988) refers to Freud's statements as "innovative" and "revolutionary" and draws from them the logical conclusion (one that had been absorbed into the culture long ago) that since, according to Freud, the sexual instinct has no built-in bond with any particular kind of object, sexual inversion is "no more than a mere difference" (p. 52), or in the current jargon, an "alternate lifestyle." Of course, by the same logic pedophilia or necrophilia are also "no more than a mere difference."

If the human sexual instinct is simply a matter of titillating sensation in the genitals and other sexually sensitive parts and the mechanical stimulation of those parts to bring about orgasm, then the desire for any object becomes difficult to explain, since masturbation would be the most immediate and most certain way of satisfying instinctual pressure. Hillman (1975), in an essay on the masturbation inhibition, posits a built-in inhibitor of masturbation as part of the sexual drive itself: "Conceding that the [masturbation] inhibition experienced in conscience as guilt anxiety is sui generis and not a cultural prohibition, perhaps its origin is biological" (p. 113). Although Hillman offers this possibility only to reject it for another thesis, his discarded conjecture is worth more serious consideration. In my view, however, he mistakes shame for guilt. Hillman cites Fenichel (1945), who, also confusing shame with guilt, writes:

In adolescence and later life, frequently not only fears and guilt feelings are still connected with masturbation, but there is even a distinct resistance on the part of the patients against enlightenment about the harmless nature of masturbation.

They seem to have some unconscious interest in believing
that masturbation is a dreadful thing. (p. 75)

Freud, in the "Introductory Lectures on Psychoanalysis"
(1917/1963), makes the statement "A phantasy of being se-
duced when no seduction has occurred is usually employed by a
child to screen the autoerotic period of his sexual activity. He
spares himself shame by retrospectively phantasizing a desired
object into those earliest times" (p. 370). It seems to me that
implied in this statement are the ideas that there is something
intrinsically shameful about masturbation and autoerotism and
that shame is a spur to sexual fantasy and the directing of libido
toward a desired object, as well as a motive for falsifying reality
by shifting responsibility for sexual pleasure to the "seducer."
    In an essay entitled "On the Universal Tendency to Debase-
ment in the Sphere of Love," Freud (1912) made the remarkable
statement "It is my belief that, however strange it may sound, we
must reckon with the possibility that something in the nature of
the sexual instinct itself is unfavorable to the realization of complete satisfaction" (pp. 188–189). Almost immediately after of-
fering this intuition he proceeded in a contradictory fashion to
blame civilization (via the incest taboo and cultural demands for
the repression of some components of the sexual instinct) for all
the constraints and inhibitions "imposed" on human sexual expression. Freud failed to develop his hunch that the human sexual
drive may have built-in constraints and inhibitions, and that his
views on the nature of the relationship between sexual regulation
and civilization might need to be turned upside down; civilization
may owe more to intrinsic constraints on sexual expression than
constraints on sexual expression owe to civilization. Had he not
backed away from his intuition Freud might have considered the
possibility that the primary built-in inhibiting, constraining, and
directing force in the complex structure of erotic life was shame.
As Schneider (1977) pointed out, Freud regarded shame in relation to sexual matters as "false" shame and prudishness, which
instigated and maintained repression, leading to a variety of neurotic symptoms and inhibitions.
    Levin (1967) expressed the view that shame was a "basic
component of the normal homeostatic mechanisms regulating the

sexual drive" (p. 270). The philosopher Max Scheler had earlier put forward the same idea in his lengthy essay on shame (written in 1913 but published posthumously in 1957, and never published in an English translation, to the best of my knowledge). Scheler argued that the human sexual drive is the conjoint product of three regulatory forces, namely, libido, shame, and sympathy. Sympathy, for Scheler, is an affective participation in the experience of another, which in the case of sexual activity is reflected in the desire to provide the other person with the same pleasure as one experiences oneself. Thus, Scheler rejected Freud's view, which identified human sexuality with libido alone. In Scheler's view the sexual drive in man is a complex self-regulating structure. To see only the libidinal component of the erotic is a biological reduction that "dehumanizes" the complex nature of human erotic life.

Scheler saw shame as a strong force opposing autoerotism and masturbation and thus serving an important "altruistic" function in socializing sexuality. Scheler believed that a true sexual instinct exists only when one begins to look for libidinal satisfaction through the intervention of another person and that it is shame, by inhibiting autoerotism, that plays the major role in the formation of the true sexual instinct.

Scheler also assigned to shame a role in the postponement of active sexual life until adequate sexual and emotional maturity has been achieved. In the young today we see a strange twist on this theme. While normally shame might, as Scheler stated, serve to delay the initiation of active sexual life, in the case of today's adolescents a variety of cultural forces undermine this important function of shame. Shame and reticence are generally negatively viewed in the world of today's adolescents. In fact, secondary shame about shame itself results in adolescents becoming sexually active at very early ages. Adolescents will often counterphobically initiate sexual activity to avoid the shame of being too ashamed to be sexually active, a trait that might result in loss of peer acceptance; it is a case of the shame of peer nonacceptance overriding the shame of sexual reticence. I personally believe that the greatly increased incidence of depression, along with a pervasive sense of hopelessness and the feeling that life has lost its meaning, which is epidemic among adolescents these days, is traceable in part to the violation of the protective function of shame in ensuring that the still psychically immature individual will not be thrown into greater physical intimacy than he or she is psychologically prepared to handle.

Emad (1972) in discussing Scheler's views on shame and sexuality noted that Scheler saw shame as operating within sexual intercourse to fulfill the following functions: "(1) it prevents attention being drawn to the anatomy and mechanism of intercourse, (2) it prevents the apperceptive isolation of sexually sensitive parts of the body from the entirety of the person, (3) under the influence of shame the sexual parts of the body are taken solely for expressional symbols of the initial affectation of the psyche (seelische Bewegung)" (p. 367). In other words, shame keeps the holistic relationship with the loved and exciting other from becoming simply a part-object affair or a matter of mechanics. Shame protects against the dissociation of the sexual act from a relationship with a whole person and inhibits the sexual impulse until the self as a whole responds to the other person in his or her wholeness; understood in this way, shame is in the service of love. As Schneider (1977) noted, to override the restraints of shame risks arousing powerful negativities, principally disgust and rage.

Recently, a patient spoke to me about a sexual encounter he had with a woman whom he was strongly sexually attracted to but otherwise disliked and devalued. He said that while they were having intercourse he found himself mentally stepping outside of the scene and observing it as though from across the room. He spoke of the disgust and revulsion he felt toward his partner in response to his heightened awareness of her sweaty fleshiness and her labored effort to satisfy herself, and also of the disgust he felt for himself.

When the sense of shame is overridden, objectification of self and other is apt to occur with accompanying shame and disgust. It might be useful to say a few words about disgust as it is understood in Tomkins's affect theory. The oral drive or hunger drive has three auxiliary lines of defense that protect the organism from ingesting noxious substances. The first line of defense is what Tomkins has labeled the affect of *dissmell*, which causes us to retract our upper lip and tilt our head up and back in an effort to distance ourselves from foul-smelling substances. Should the first line of defense fail and we take into our mouth something spoiled or noxious that is bad-tasting, the affect of disgust is called into play and we spit out the noxious substance. Should that protective mechanism fail, then nausea followed by vomiting becomes the next line of defense. The object of disgust is the prototypical ambivalently held object, attractive and desirable enough to be brought into close contact but then rejected as noxious.

The sense of shame prevents the libidinal component of the sexual drive from leading us into closer intimacy with another than is compatible with our emotional readiness for such an encounter. When the sense of shame is overridden, and sexual contact with the other is made regardless of our readiness, the situation becomes an analogue of the oral disgust situation and the same affect is apt to be aroused, resulting in disgust toward the objectified other and oneself. Schneider (1977) examines this phenomenon more fully in his insightful study of shame, where the interested reader may pursue this theme in greater depth.

Freud's writings reveal his basic assumption that instinctual man is the natural man and that the superego is, both historically and developmentally, a later-appearing structure (derived from the oedipal complex) that conceals from man his true nature through repression of his natural tendencies. According to Freud, the affects that instigate and maintain that repression are shame, guilt, and disgust. Hence, Freud concluded that if we aim to acquaint someone with his natural, true self, we cannot allow the person's shame to deter us from that task. Psychoanalysis thus became "shameless" in its relentless pursuit of the repressed.

Scheler says that shame may operate in three different ways with respect to instinctual stirrings. Shame may act to inhibit the movement of libido and prevent the *formation* of a complex of ideas, images, and desires; the complex is nipped in the bud, so to speak. Or if this complex is *already formed*, shame may appear after the fact and instigate repression. Or the individual may feel shame only if there is a threat of exposure to the negative judgement of others; here suppression and concealment, rather than repression are apt to be called into play.

In the first manner of operation, mentioned in the preceding paragraph, shame is *not* a repressive force, as Freud perceived it to be in general. Shame, having nipped the complex in the bud and thus prevented its formation, obviates any need for repression. Shame is in this instance not an affective reaction to something already present but an anticipation or presentiment of a possible future development; it corresponds with what we have called the "sense of shame." Scheler speculated that the hysterics whom Freud treated, and who provided him with the material on which he based his theory of the sexual etiology of neurosis, suffered from a moribund or overpowered sense of shame and consequently were unable to check in their germinal form the ideas and desires corresponding to libidinal stirrings of various kinds; instead, such desires proliferated luxuriantly and became dominating psychic configurations that then evoked shame affect, which in turn instigated repression.

Let us return to Freud's (1905/1953) conclusion that "the sexual instinct is in the first instance independent of its object; nor is its origin likely to be due to its objects attractions" (p. 148). If sexual drive is primarily a matter of physiology and only secondarily a psychic event, then Freud's position follows logically from that assumption. From the sleep laboratories has come the knowledge that cycles of dreaming are accompanied by penile erection. Since the activation of the sexual drive during sleep is accompanied by dream imagery, it is not unlikely that the activation of the sexual drive during wakefulness is also accompanied on the unconscious level by the activation of a highly abstract archetypal representation of the opposite gender in the heterosexual population or the same gender in the homosexual population. These archetypal activations would then lead to a search in memory, in creative fantasy, or in the everyday world of other living beings for acceptable representatives of the archetype. The poet W. B. Yeats recognized the power of the archetype in the sexual drive:

> Eternity is passion, girl or boy
> Cry at the onset of sexual joy
> "For ever and for ever"; then awake
> Ignorant what Dramatis Personae spake.
> (Whence had they come?)

If shame inhibits masturbation, then the pursuit of the arche-typal other in masturbatory fantasy will produce shame anxiety, worry, and hypochondriacal brooding and thus favor the pursuit of the archetype in the form of the real, living, flesh and blood other. According to the theory I am presenting here, the sexual drive, in its wholeness, consists of a set of physiological mecha-nisms plus the psychological activation of highly abstract arche-typal "images" plus the sense of shame that inhibits the exclu-sively autoerotic use of these images, exerts psychological pressure for the selection of the best available representative or manifestation of the archetype, inhibits premature sexual union, and promotes sexual love.

Personal, biographical, and cultural factors will obviously influence the process of selecting the person who will be consid-ered the best available embodiment of the archetypal representa-tion associated with the sexual drive. Looked at in the way I have outlined, the sexual instinct is a psychophysiological structure and, from this point of view, an instinct that is *not* strictly independent of its object. If it were independent of its object, deviations in the choice of object would be the rule and would not even be recognized as deviations.

So we come to the conclusion that Freud's theory of psy-chosexual development was not *psycho*sexual enough. As Schimek (1987) said of Freud, "As a 19th-century positivist, he believed that mental processes had only a kind of borrowed reality which had to be ultimately grounded on material events and processes as the only true reality (bodily stimulation by the mother in infancy, prehistoric events, physiological basis of drives, etc.)" (p. 962).

Freud (1905/1953) wrote that "experience of the cases that are considered abnormal has shown us that in them the sexual instinct and the sexual object are merely soldered together" (p.148). Had he stopped at this point there would be no problem. His next move was typical Freud; he extrapolated from the study of the abnormal to the universal and went on to say, "We are thus warned to loosen the bond that exists in our thought between instinct and object. It seems probable that the sexual instinct is in the first instance independent of its object; nor is its origin likely to be due to its object's attractions" (p. 148). One is not logically entitled to conclude that because the study of "cases that are considered abnormal" suggests that in these conditions the sexual instinct and the sexual object are merely soldered together, instinct and object are therfore soldered together in all cases.

It is but a short step indeed from the idea that instinct and object are "in the first instance" independent to a determination to make that theoretical independence into actual independence. Is there not a chillingly imperative quality to Freud's statement "We are thus warned to loosen the bond that exists in our thought between instinct and object?" Has the voice of the castrating father found unrecognized expression in Freud's prose? We are vaguely threatened—"warned" to loosen the connection in our thought (in our mind, in our behavior) between instinct and object. Western culture has taken this Freudian imperative seriously.

Let us again join Leslie Farber (1976) in his scathing commentary on the Masters and Johnson research project investigating the nature of the female orgasm. Commenting that the project itself interested him more than the findings, he explains why:

> It strikes me as one of those occasional yet remarkable enterprises that, despite their creators' intentions, quite transcend their original and modest scientific boundaries, so as to become vivid allegories of our present dilemma, containing their own images of man—while at the same time charting a New Jerusalem for our future. . . . part of the power of the enterprise as constitutive symbol must be credited to the director's unflagging lack of imagination and his passionate naiveté, which stay undeterred by all the proprieties, traditions, and accumulated wisdom that would only complicate his course. (pp. 128–129)

As most reader know, Masters and Johnson's primary investigative tool was the motion picture camera with which they filmed their female "subjects" bringing themselves to orgasm through masturbation, in the laboratory setting, at presumably scheduled times, in the presence of the investigative and filming crew.

Since prostitutes were ruled out as not constituting a "normal" sample, subjects were chosen from among medical students and medical students' wives who volunteered and were paid a modest fee for participating in the project. In speculating about what qualities an ideal subject for such an experiment would have, Farber (1976) writes,

> In a general way, her sexuality would have to be autonomous, separate from and unaffected by her ordinary world. "World" here would have to include not only affection but all those exigencies of human existence which tend to shape our erotic possibilities. Objectively, her sexuality would be mechanically accessible or "on call" under circumstances which would be, if not intimidating, at least distracting to most bodies; hers would have to be indifferent to the entire range of experiences, pleasant and unpleasant, whose claim is not only not salacious but makes us forget there is such a thing as sexuality. Her lust would lie to hand, ready to be invoked and consummated, in sickness or in health, in coitus or "automanipulation," in homosexuality or heterosexuality, in exasperation or calm, hesitancy or certainty, playfulness or despair. (p. 134)

How's that for independence of instinct from object and freedom from shame? Farber ironically refers to such a woman as "the latter-day Queen of Courtly Love," the dream of modern men, and the envy of "less fortunate" modern women. So we see how far we have taken Freud's injunction.

Farber asks, How does all of this affect those of us who could not hope to qualify for this research, either as volunteers or as scientists? He ruefully concludes that since the findings of sexology are all in the public domain or potentially so, we turn our bedrooms into our own poor laboratories, where we impose on our bodies whatever the most current scientific research has "discovered" about sex. It is out of our bodies' failure to meet these imperatives that we form our vision of the ideal experience.

It was also fitting that the motion picture camera was the principal investigative tool in the Masters and Johnson project, since the camera is the leading symbol of the triumph of objectification in the modern era, a theme we will develop at greater length in Chapter 10. Barfield (1977) noted, "It used to be said that the camera cannot lie. But in fact it always does lie. Just because it looks only in that immediate way, the camera looks always at and never into what it sees" (p. 73). The literalist might object that Masters and Johnson's camera not only looked at but into its subjects, noting that a specially designed phallus-like camera photographed vaginal secretions," droplets," and "engorgements"—but, then, only a literalist mentality could have conceived of the project in the first place. If one holds the view that shame, and the sense of shame as it affects human sexuality, is only an undesirable obstacle to a liberated and "healthy" sexual life, then the sense of shame should not only be eliminated from the bedroom but from the scientific laboratory as well.

Farber (1976) noted with regard to sex that

> its particular difference from everything else in this life lies in the possibility that sex offers man for regaining *his own* body through knowing the body of his loved one. Should he fail that *knowing* and *being known*, should he lapse into all those ways of *knowing about* which he had proudly learned to confuse with *knowing*—both bodies will again escape him. (p. 127)

What Farber is getting at, in my view, is the difference between the truly erotic—as an I–thou communicative mode, protected by shame, in which neither other or self is objectified—and the narrowly sexual, as a disjunctive, objectifying experience. The distinction between the erotic and the narrowly sexual is not to be found in Freud. Straus (1980) said of shame: "It does not constrain the erotic, as is assumed in psychoanalysis, but makes the erotic possible for the first time" (p. 222).

The myth of Psyche and Eros is instructive in this regard. As the reader will recall, Eros, or Cupid, was the son of Venus. Psyche, the youngest daughter of a king, was so beautiful that people ceased to worship Venus. Venus, narcissistically injured and enraged, sent her son Eros to make Psyche fall in love with the ugliest creature he could find. However, when Eros saw Psyche he fell in love with her himself and could not obey his mother's command. He arranged for Psyche to be whisked away on the breezes to a palace with jeweled gates and golden doors, where she was waited on by unseen hands. At night when she went to bed she was joined in the darkness by Eros in human form. He told her that he was her husband and that she would enjoy the happiest of lives if only she would refrain from seeking to find out who he was or trying to see him. She began to love him deeply. Nevertheless, after a while, she became somewhat lonely for her family and asked that her sisters be allowed to visit her. Eros reluctantly agreed and had them brought over on the next breeze. The sisters were filled with envy when they saw her situation. When they learned that Psyche had never seen her husband, they terrified her into believing he might be a monster. Torn between the warnings of her husband and the expressed fears of her sisters, Psyche gave in to her curiosity and fear; when she next went to bed for the night, she took a lantern and dagger with her. After Eros had fallen asleep, she lit the lamp and held it to his face, raising the dagger to slay him should he be a monster. When she saw the beautiful features of the god, Psyche was so startled that she let a drop of hot oil from the lamp fall on Eros and he awoke. Realizing that Psyche had violated his prohibition, Eros arose and flew away.

While acknowledging that myths lend themselves to many interpretations, I am nevertheless inclined to interpret the myth as pointing to a vital relationship between erotic love and the sense of shame. The erotic must remain veiled and the claims of shame must be respected. One must not aggressively objectify the other and try to see all or know all about the beloved, for such shameless intrusiveness will cause love to flee. Erotic love is made up of libido plus archetypal activation plus a sense of shame plus shared consciousness. The burning lamp in the myth has a double significance: The flaming oil gives light that reveals, but that exposure to the aggressive, objectifying gaze of the other is accompanied by sense of violation and the reddening burn of shame.

·9·

Embracing Objecthood

John Berger (1977) has written about the way men view women and the way women have traditionally viewed themselves. Acknowledging that significant shifts have been taking place in this regard, he nevertheless believes that it is still largely true that:

> A man's presence is dependent upon the promise of power which he embodies. . . . A man's presence suggests what he is capable of doing to you or for you. . . . By contrast, a woman's presence expresses her own attitude to herself, and defines what can and cannot be done to her. . . . From earliest childhood she has been taught and persuaded to survey herself continually. . . . She has to survey everything she is and everything she does because how she appears to others and ultimately how she appears to men, is of crucial importance for what is normally thought of as the success of her life. Her own sense of being in herself is supplanted by a sense of being appreciated as herself by another. . . . Men look at women. Women watch themselves being looked at. This determines not only most relations between men and women but also the relation of women to themselves. The surveyor of woman in herself is male,: the surveyed, female. Thus she turns herself into an object—and most particularly an object of vision: a sight. (pp. 46–47)

Although turning oneself into an object is by no means an exclusively feminine enterprise, Berger is right in suggesting that the cultural pressures on females to so regard themselves is apt to be greater than any similar pressure on males. To the extent

121

that one has turned oneself into an object for others, an object of vision, one risks having the clinical label of narcissistic or hysterical or histrionic personality applied to oneself. This is so because it is the nature of hysteria that aesthetic considerations become dominant over other considerations. According to Leslie Farber (1976), the aestheticism of hysteria is concerned with many variations on two questions: "Am I pretty?" (or "Am I manly?") and "Am I bright?" Combined, they produce the question, "Am I interesting?" or "Do you like me?"

Stoller (1979) has published material from interviews with a person to whom he assigned the pseudonym Olympia. She makes her living as a stripper, centerfold model, and starlet. She was interviewed for the purpose of being presented to a medical school class as a prototypical specimen of the female hysteric— or histrionic personality, as she is now more fashionably called. This interview material provides a means of "fleshing out" (pun intended) some of the theoretical considerations of the preceding chapters. (Portions of the interviews have been deleted at those places indicated by asterisks.)

INTERVIEWS

S: Tell me about yourself.

O: O.K. One thing I have to my advantage is that I am totally without shame. Nothing shocks me, surprises me, or embarrasses me. I can be very blunt and very honest. Someone can ask me anything and be very direct with me; it never bothers me or offends me. [These statements are now being rattled off almost as a set speech, the speech of a star being interviewed for the hundredth time: to give the effect of normality, competence, breathless enthusiasm, earnestness, intelligence, and professionalism.] I'm trying to establish myself as a sexual star and have been working to create my skills as a sexual type of entertainer. I've paid a lot of attention to observing what a person's response is in entertainment. You don't decide what an audience wants: rather you fill a void that's there. I try to keep myself receptive to what they want to see and keep myself as archetypal [a nice word for a fetish] as possible, to say a little about

122

myself in each thing I do so that each person in the audience will see what they want to see. I've always been fascinated with go-go. Because what I'm really fascinated with is dance. Nude dancing is the most credible dance form, because you're actually doing something that makes sense: there's no beginning, middle, and end with a story being told. Everybody knows what you're doing. Lots of times dancing loses credibility because it looks like a bunch of fruits prancing around. But I am interested in my dancing because of the sexualism in it. From what I've seen, sex really does rule the world on all levels. That seems to be the strongest thing in any human—that sexual drive. My choreographer told me one time, "We have a lot of work to do; cut out your sex life completely so we can rechannel your energy." It was true. We progressed about four years in six months. My interest in go-go dancing started from about five years old. I can remember standing on a pillow and doing burlesque routines. There wasn't a drawer in my room that wasn't broken from taking it out and standing on it until my feet went through. Then I would build huge colossal things from upside-down chairs and tables and drawers on top of the bed. Then I would strip. Or sometimes sing. There wasn't an audience. I'd do it myself. The reason I like working on stage is to create illusions and fantasies. I do that for myself. And it's nice if an audience can share them too, because I'm getting appreciation for the illusions. But mainly I do it for myself. I don't think it's exhibitionism because I don't feel naked when I have my clothes off. Instead, I have always thought it was that I was entertaining people. The major reason I don't feel naked is because I'm confidant with my figure. I can go up on stage and take all my clothes off and feel just as comfortable as I do right now. But if I had to go up on stage and tell my deepest personal secrets, that would make me feel naked. But not my body. There are millions of versions of it. All women have the same equipment I have.

All the time I was growing up, my mother said, "Aren't you ever going to learn to sit like a lady? We're so tired of looking at your underwear," never realizing that would be my fortune. All the random incidents in my life, all the people I've known, everything that's happened ties into now. Just recently, someone told me that he's never seen anyone so happy in his life.

My memory goes way back. My first memory was [at] six

months. In the memory, I don't remember my mother; I don't remember myself; there's no people; there's no action. All I remember is the bathroom. With all those early memories: no event and no people.

I remember when I was around four, whenever I had to tinkle, my father'd take me to the men's room, because he didn't think I'd be safe in the ladies' room by myself. I remember standing by the urinals, watching all the men tinkle; that was one of my favorite forms of entertainment. He and my mother believed that children wouldn't be safe going into a public rest room by themselves: if you sent a four-year-old kid into the ladies' room by herself, you don't know who might be in there. There might be some kind of sex crime, for instance. My mother had pointed out to me in the newspaper where little boys had gone into the rest room at gas stations and had their peepies cut off by some razor-wielding fiend who's hiding out in there. I don't think they were as concerned about a sex crime as much as the permanent mutilation involved with it. They're both very, very naive: they were sure that in public rest rooms, if you send a child in by themselves, there is always the possibility that a mutilating homicidal maniac is waiting.

S: Even in the ladies room?

* * *

O: I have only been engaged once. Because I don't think it's for me. I don't like making sacrifices for an involvement I would have to make: I wouldn't want to ever cancel a dancing lesson or anything. Because my business is to model, sing, act, and dance. They all fall in the category of entertainment and the trick is to make them all work together. I've developed an incredibly close relationship with people who are involved in it—my manager, my choreographer, my dancing teacher, singing teacher, the woman who draws up the advertising work that I use in the trades, the songwriter, the costume maker, my photographer, the guy who writes up biographies on me and publicity releases and lines that I should drop in certain situations. Oh—and a financial backer. We're all involved in the same thing—creating a certain sexual image. And they're as much a part of that image. I remove myself from myself. I see myself as a commodity. They are as much me as I am. We're all equal pieces of the pie. All I am is the physical likeness in the act. Without them I would be nothing.

S: Who are you?

O: The real me doesn't have a name, doesn't have a face. It doesn't have that spark of life or whatever.

S: The person who goes by the name of Olympia is not you exactly, is that right?

O: No, because they haven't named. They've named my body, my [public] personality. It's hard to understand because there aren't words to describe it.

* * *

S: So you look on yourself—on Olympia—as a corporation, in which different people do different things? Your contribution is to put your body out there—

O: Yes, because the physical is the instrument by which the performance is put on. Entertainers aren't born, they are created. All entertainers are put together. And I do have someone who's put me together: my manager. He tells me how to dress, what style of makeup, just everything. If I weren't put together, I never could have cared less about my physical appearance. As a result, I looked very, very dumpy because I didn't have any identity. As a child I never had any kind of image or appearance. Just to live. Then I realized if I was going to succeed, I'd have to be put together. I am trying to establish myself as a particular personality. That's what's nice about *Raunch*. Though I plan to play a part, the reader doesn't know that. They think that's me and that's my name. So now, I have much more credibility with people. I say things and people listen now, even though I'm exactly the same person I was five years ago. The main centerfold is saying that. So it must be important. I had a terrible problem as a teenager; there was a terrible waste occurring. There was no way I could reach millions of people so that they would say, "Yes. She did brush her hair today!" (laughs) I've always needed to be a legend.

125

So I got right down to business. I started pushing. It worked. I was able to get parts in films. I started dancing. When I first started I was really terrible. But I realized if I let talent stand in my way, I would never accomplish it. Everyone admitted I was the worst dancer they had ever seen. And no one could imagine how anyone had that much nerve to stand up there and dance when they were so awful. But I had a huge following, and I was making a fortune in tips, I tried so hard. Go-go.

When the man who is now my choreographer came in the first time and saw me, he realized that he couldn't find a bigger challenge: there was never going to be a worse dancer. It was like Pygmalion. I became the best dancer there. I sit in the kitchen with my choreographer, and the guy that writes up the things for me, and the woman in the advertising; we sat there and decided, now what is my personality going to be? We decide it will be this and that, but we leave the space open, trying to make it as archetypal as possible. What type of speech, what kind of walk, what's her childhood, what affects a certain demographic but not another demographic? The same way you market any product; the same way as this cigarette. The same way you market a package of cigarettes, we are marketing sexual personality. A person that appeals to the sexuality in everyone.

S: Are you interested in sex for yourself or only as a product?

O: Oh, I have the same desires as everyone. But at this stage of the game, I feel that sex only takes away that same hour that I would be on the phone to my costume maker, for instance. I barely have enough time to sleep and eat as it is. I don't have the time. When I do have the time—and who knows when that will be, maybe in a year—I have the same desires everyone does.

The sexuality in me extends in all areas of my life, particularly creativity. I write a bit, and I'm a big fan of science fiction. And I realized one day that the biggest part of the female sex organs, the most important and best part, isn't what's there, but what isn't. It's the space, it's the void. I was thinking about how all women don't have the same fears of actual physical inadequacies that men do: it's what's not there that counts, not what *is* there. Wouldn't it be interesting [science fiction story she may write] if there were a linkup, that people are linked up to everything in nature? Like a

126

black hole in space so that on the day that a black hole in space became activated and began to suck up the whole universe, all the vaginas in the world also became activated to sucking to a lesser extent: pulling up the carpets, the little knickknacks, and all of them turn themselves inside out and disappear.

* * *

S: What is the biggest visual turn on you've ever had?

O: It's the one wearing the mask. Because there's a uniqueness about it. And it's anonymous. A mask of some kind: I was wearing one and they were wearing one. I was always wanting to do something different with him. So we decided to wear masks; we both agreed there was an appeal in it. No matter how free you are with another person, you're aware they are watching you—your expressions, what you're doing. But when your face is covered, you don't have to worry what shows on your face. And there's no point in looking at the other person's face because it is covered. So it's just pure physical pleasure for pleasure's sake—anonymousness. And you couldn't do the same in black darkness, because you would not be able to see the body. You have to mask facial expressions. Just a mask to cover up. I tried with eyes covered. But that is no good, because then you can't see out and see the other's body. The mask should just hide facial expressions: the other person's facial expressions, and [so] that they can't see yours. Sometimes you might feel a particular way, but you have to force a big smile for your partner's sake, for their security. With a mask, you're freer.

* * *

O: I don't know if you've ever tried this: I have a boyfriend with a videotape setup. It was terrific. It's really nice to be able to watch what you were just experiencing. There is something about photographing it that made it more enjoyable than plain watching it. I could see what I was doing and tried to work on it and get it better. Things like "Gee. Next time, I'm taking my underwear off." Or, "I'll pull my hair up from now on; look how raggedy the ends are."

127

That's picking up the little things, but basically it's fun to watch actual sex activities.

S: Are you ever dissatisfied with your performance?

O: Oh, yeah. If it's a bad camera angle and if the camera isn't moving, you have to move in front of it. You get something which at one angle would be quite lovely. But you get in a bad angle: I might look a little bit cruddy.

S: When there is no camera and you are having sexual relations, are you still on camera?

O: Yes. I'm on camera twenty-four hours a day. I never felt attached to my body. I felt I would have much more freedom as a part of the collective unconscious, as a spirit, if I were freed of the physical limitations in a container like this [body]. Without the container, I could totally disperse and be in a billion places all over the universe at the same time. But it's not just a container; it's a tool for accomplishing things. It helps us to physically identify ourselves to other people. And we decorate the outside when we dress, style ourselves, carry ourselves. When we dress ourselves and when we carry ourselves, we can give any kind of appearance we like. That's why female impersonators are usually much more feminine and put together than actual women, because women just take for granted since they are a female body. Whereas a female impersonator will study all the feminine movements and style of dress.

S: Did you study that?

O: Yes. I've studied all that.

S: Are you a female impersonator?

O: Yes. Because I'm a natural clod. I feel that I'm a female impersonator. I like to joke because I don't have that natural femininity. My coach told me: why don't I try a wig on? So I put my wig on and come to class. It would be crooked on my head with a point up at the end and the bangs hanging down in front, my eyelashes up to here, my nail polish smeared all over. None of those things that seem to come so naturally to some women ever came naturally to me. I always thought I had the grace of a truck driver but I discovered that it's not a matter of gracefulness, it's a matter of knowing how to do things by studying. For example, I could show you two ways of sitting on the floor, one graceful like an accomplished dancer and one like a clod.

S: Which would be you?

O: Hopefully, the studied one.

S: But that implies it's not you.

O: But it's an accomplishment. What purpose am I here for, if not my accomplishments?

S: *Who are you?*

O: Who? Olympia Dancing-Doll: The Sweet with the SuperSupreme.

S: What the hell is that?

O: That's the title of my act. And all the years they told me, wouldn't I ever learn to sit right, they were so sick of looking at my underwear. And it came to be my fortune, at least with *Raunch*. But it's always in the same poses I was in as a kid.

S: So you have an unfair advantage.

O: Lewdity comes naturally to me. Lewdness for lewdness' sake.

S: You don't look that way now. Am I missing something or is the "lewdity" an act?

O: Oh. The lewdity is an act; that's why I do it. I become bored very, very easily.

S: Have you ever in your life been real?

O: No. Because everything I do I can see as part of a movie scene. When I go to the grocery store, it is act 1, scene 3: "At the grocery store." It's not, I just went to the grocery store. It is either in a film or on stage or something I will eventually write.

S: So even now, when you're on stage with an actual television camera here, there's another stage on which this is taking place.

O: Yes. What else!

S: Is there ever a moment when a feeling slips through that has not been observed or studied or controlled or planned?

O: I don't think so. When I was growing up, my father would say, "Look at it this way. Imagine how good it's going to look in your autobiography." So I got used to thinking in terms of everything being written.

S: [I point at her] This is a body. Is it your body?

O: Yes.

S: Are you your body?

O: No. I'm not my body but it is my body.

S: How does it feel inside your body? You are inside your body. Am I wording it right?

O: No, I'm not inside it. The actual me is just different degrees of energy. As far as a body, a personality, a voice, and a mental process is concerned, they are for me to make use of. They are something for the energy force to propel for the sake of actions. So I am "The Sweet with the SuperSupreme." "Strip the Starlet": that's the name of my act. (pp. 72–82)

What are we to make of Olympia's opening "proud" claim to be "totally without shame" in the light of what follows? Obviously, like a great many members of Western society, she considers shamelessness desirable. To be without shame seems to be one of the primary goals of her life; how well she has succeeded and at what price becomes clearer as she talks about herself and her life. There are many indications of significant shame experiences in her earlier life, such as her recollections of being shamed for presumably unself-conscious bodily exposure (e.g., "And all the years they told me wouldn't I ever learn to sit right, they were so sick of looking at my underwear"). For Olympia public nudity is not shame inducing partly because she has defensively dissociated her sense of self from her body ("What's so different about my body? There are billions of versions of it . . . I see my body as a tool, something to be used") and partly because nudity can be a form of dress, as I shall elaborate upon a little later. If shame is triggered by the experience of being objectified by the other while wanting to be related in an intersubjective mode, then the painful discrepancy can be removed by embracing objecthood and renouncing one's claims as a subject, a solution that replaces the self with a constructed persona and replaces spontaneous personal responsiveness with cultivated and rehearsed performance.

Despite her dissociation of her sense of self from her body (a very respectable Cartesian dissociation), Olympia can conceive of some aspects of her experience as so intimately bound to her sense of self (however tenuous that sense of self might be) that the public exposure of such "secrets" would evoke shame.

Olympia claims the right of being pure subject when she hides her face by wearing a mask during intercourse—her biggest visual "turn on." Because the face is the display board of the affects and the bodily site where the self is most localized, it is more difficult to dissociate one's sense of self from the face than from other parts of the body. In fact, the display of the body may serve to distract the viewer from the face and may thus, to some degree, protect the facial self from objectification and render the person less vulnerable to shame. A singer who had to appear unclothed in the stage production *O Calcutta* noted to her surprise that her performance anxiety (i.e., shame anxiety) decreased. She stated, "They would be so busy looking at my breasts, they wouldn't notice my performance" (cited in Plaut, 1990). The use of heavy facial makeup by "sexual performers" of all sorts also serves as a mask to conceal the presence of the subjective self.

Stoller refers to Olympia as displaying signs and symptoms of "identity diffusion." I believe her to be caught in what Lichtenstein (1963) referred to as the dilemma of identity.

> the subjective experience of ourselves as existing individuals is not compatible with our attempts to conceptualize this experience. When we talk about ourselves, we attempt to deal with ourselves as if we were, as Hannah Arendt calls it, a "what." But being a "who," we are not properly capable of looking on ourselves as a "what." In doing it the "who" quality of our inner experience is lost. (p. 174)

131

Olympia seems to understand this quite well. When Stoller asks, '' The person who goes by the name of Olympia is not you exactly, is that right?'', she answers, "No, because they haven't named . They've named my body, my [public] personality. Its hard to understand because there aren't words to describe it." If there are words to describe the self, those words and that description would belong to the realm of objective self-awareness; they would be about a what instead of a who. The subjective sense of self is thus ineffable. Olympia forgets her own insight that "there aren't words to describe it" and goes on to talk about being a part of the collective unconscious. When she talks about how as the performer Olympia she has been put together by her manager she is reported as saying

O: He tells me how to dress, what style of makeup, just everything. If I weren't put together, *I never really could have cared less about my physical appearance. As a result, I looked very, very dumpy because I didn't have any identity. As a child, I* never had any kind of image or appearance. Just to live." [emphasis mine]

In the unedited transcript of the interview this portion went as follows:

O: And I do have someone who's put me together, my manager, tells me how to dress, what style of makeup, just everything.

S: What would you be like if you weren't together?

O: If I weren't *put* together? *I never really could have cared less about my physical appearance. So as a result I looked very, very dumpy cause I didn't take identity with it.* I would be wearing the most loose clothing, most comfortable I could find, probably wrinkled and dirty and torn. And it wouldn't matter if I had a million dollars, I'd still look like a bum. I would be barefoot. If I wouldn't be arrested, I'd just walk around naked. The only reason I would put anything on at all is so I wouldn't be arrested. But *as a child I wanted nothing more than to live wild as a hermit in the mountains and never brush my hair, never brush my teeth, never get dressed, never have*

132

any kind of image or appearance. Just take it all for granted, just live."

It is quite apparent that in the edited version of this portion of the interview the meaning of her statements has been significantly, albeit unintentionally, altered. In the unedited version she seems to be saying that if she hadn't acquiesced in becoming an object, that is, in being put together by someone else, she would have lived the life of Nature's child, with her indwelling sense of self, and unconcerned about image or appearance— clearly her notion of a happier state of existence. Not identifying oneself with one's physical appearance is a very different thing from not having an identity. It is also interesting to note that her comments illustrate two different forms or modes of being undressed, a distinction drawn by John Berger (1977). There is nakedness, which is unself-conscious and natural, and there is nudity, which is a presentation of oneself as an object. Berger (1977) in his essay on the nude in Western art observed:

> To be naked is to be oneself.
> To be nude is to be seen naked by others and yet not recognized for oneself. A naked body has to be seen as an object in order to become a nude. (The sight of it as an object stimulates the use of it as an object.) Nakedness reveals itself. Nudity is placed on display.
> To be naked is to be without disguise.
> To be on display is to have the surface of one's own skin, the hairs of one's own body, turned into a disguise which in that situation can never be discarded. The nude is condemned to never being naked. Nudity is a form of dress. (p. 54)

Thus, it is not really so strange that a nude dancer should long for true nakedness. Olympia also displays the kind of "camera consciousness" that makes her life seem like a succession of movie scenes. We will have more to say about camera consciousness in the next chapter.

Olympia's situation is more sensational and dramatic than that of most late 20th-century Western females, but certain commonalities are not difficult to identify. The "average" woman (and to a lesser extent, the "average" man) is also, to a great extent, a corporate product; her managers are the ad agencies, the fashion industry, and the Media. The aim is the same: to make her an agreeable object (or "fetish," to use Stoller's term) and to persuade her that her only hope of happiness lies in her acquiescence to them and their "benevolent" intentions and interests.

A women in her late 20s, who came for treatment with the complaint "I can't seem to be faithful to my husband," tried to encourage her husband to consider a sexual encounter with a woman friend of his from his office. She also recalled that on one occasion, when she had had a couple of drinks, she offered her husband's services to one of her divorced girlfriends who had made a comment about missing sex. Although she recognized that she might be trying to relieve her guilt over her extramarital activities, this did not seem to be the most pressing motive for her suggestion. She thought it would be interesting to watch them make love (not so much out of strong voyeuristic interests—she claimed to be turned off by porno films) to see if her husband "looked as good" making love to someone else as she experienced him to be when he made love to her. She wanted objectivity and distance. Only if she felt that her husband would be considered a desirable lover by other females and by herself as objective observer could she conceive of the possibility of really valuing him, maybe loving him, and perhaps not being so easily drawn into extramarital encounters. She recognized that she had been drawn into an unsatisfying sexual relationship with her boss because she knew that many other women in the office found him attractive. Determining who was desirable became, for her, a matter of taking a head count. Like a great many people, she operated on the principle that the more people there are who consider you desirable the more desirable you are—a principle essential to a successfully functioning consumer society.

· 10 ·

Shamelessness and Modern Society

The fabulous Greeks made of shame a goddess—Aidos. She was the source of dignity, decency, and good manners. An offense committed against Aidos was avenged by the goddess Nemesis. Long live shame!

ERIC HOFFER (1974)

A major part of the Freudian legacy is a general cultural disrespect for shame. Freud's failure, and the failure of later psychoanalysts, to recognize shame's healthy functions led to the culturally disastrous notion that freedom from shame (including the sense of shame) is the mark of the healthy personality. The effects of this disrespect for the legitimate claims of shame are all around us. One major effect is that, as Farber observed, sex has lost its viability as a human experience over the last 50 to 60 years. Also witness the general shamelessness and corruption of our public officials and the leaders in the financial and corporate world as well as the ever-increasing tawdriness, vulgarity, and tastelessness of the entertainment products offered to us. The pop culture heroes offered the young—in films, on TV, and on the rock music scene—are mostly noteworthy for their pride in their aggressiveness, crudity, narcissism, and general boorishness—traits that would have been cause for shame in former times. We have for many years now been witnessing a kind of moral inversion in our society in which some of the sorriest specimens of humanity are lionized and idolized. The press, piously championing the public's right to know, knows no sense of shame in its intrusion into the private lives of anyone and everyone, pandering to a morbid public voyeurism. Many people believe that relationships between men and women in Western societies are at an all-time low; to the extent that this is true, could it not have something to do with the fact that when the sense of shame is lost or devalued, Eros flees, as he has in our times?

Hoffer (1974) wrote:

> Our intellectual mentors strive to infect us with a sense of guilt—about Vietnam, the negro, the poor, pollution—and frown on shame as reactionary and repressive. But whether or not a sense of guilt will make us a better people, the loss of shame threatens our survival as a civilized society. For most of the acts we are ashamed of are not punishable by law, and civilized living depends on the observance of unenforceable rules. (p. 10)

Shamelessness has been a recurrent problem in the history of civilizations. Thucydides might as well have been speaking about our times when he had this to say about the demoralization of the Greek states during the Peloponnesian War:

> Proper shame is now termed sheer stupidity: shamelessness on the other hand is called manliness: voluptuousness passes for good tone: haughtiness for good education: lawlessness for freedom: honourable dealing is dubbed hypocrisy, and dishonesty, good fortune. (as cited in Barfield, 1985, p. 162)

Lowenfeld (1976), a psychoanalyst writing on the subject of shamelessness, offers the following assessment of the reduction of the sense of shame in regard to sexual matters:

> The decline of shame in the attitude toward sex, *while it confused the lives of many people and endangered the quality of love*, also enriched and freed the libido from unnecessary chains. In all other (nonsexual) respects, shamelessness can

hardly be seen as anything but a decline in civilized living. (pp. 68–69, emphasis mine)

Lowenfeld's paper is interesting in that he derives the increasing societal shamelessness in nonsexual matters from the decline in shame associated with sexual matters. The argument follows familiar Freudian lines and goes as follows: Shame has its genesis in childhood as a defense against pregenital and genital drives, but later in its development the sense of shame acquires enlarged meanings and functions in upholding the structure of society. Shame thus acquires a relative and fragile functional independence while maintaining genetic continuity with the component sexual drives. The functional independence of shame is vulnerable to being undermined when the original drive components that shame served to defend against are allowed freer expression, as they have been in contemporary society, where exhibitionistic and voyeuristic drives are freely indulged. Eliminate shame in the sexual area and, Lowenfeld concludes, the larger societal values that are upheld by an extended and displaced sense of shame are in jeopardy. The whole structure of civilized society is thus a house of cards precariously balanced on shame as defense against components of the sexual drive. Interestingly, if this line of reasoning were valid, it would constitute one of the strongest arguments against pornography and for a certain level of censorship and societal repressiveness with regard to sexual mores.

Although I have already discussed the limitations of the Freudian conceptions of the nature of shame and I reject the idea of deriving the general sense of shame from exclusively sexual sources, must we therefore dismiss the relationship between general shamelessness and sexual shamelessness that Lowenfeld points to? We sense that Lowenfeld is onto something and that there is indeed some important relationship here, even if we don't subscribe to the orthodox Freudian explanation of that relationship. As I noted earlier, Straus (1980) has contested the notion that voyeurism and exhibitionism are normal components of the sexual drive, and he has argued that they reflect an alteration in communicative mode, involving distancing and objectification. If the function of shame (more accurately, the sense of shame) is to defend against exhibitionism and voyeurism, as many psychoanalysts have insisted, then by implication shame defends against objectification and distancing in personal relations. The role of the sense of shame in defending against objectification and distancing is not recognized in psychoanalytic theorizing. If voyeurism and exhibitionism are rampant in our society, it seems to me attributable to a more general breakdown in restrictions against objectification of others.

Capitalism has always been based on objectification of workers and consumers; if we are to understand modern shamelessness, we have to take into account the fact that modern capitalism has conjoined objectification, greed, and sexuality as the prime movers of the economic system.

In *Intimate Matters: A History of Sexuality in America*, D'Emilio and Freedman (1988) write the following:

> For almost two centuries sexuality has been moving into the marketplace. At first largely restricted to prostitution and located in a marginally urban underworld out of view of the middle class, sex gradually became the province of big time entrepreneurs and pervaded the entire culture. The concert salons of the nineteenth century and the dance halls of the Progressive era were the prototypes of the elaborate high-tech disco; the titillating postcards and one-reelers of the turn of the century were but pale forerunners of the glossy sex magazines and feature-length video cassettes of the 1980s. However, not only did modern capitalism sell sexual fantasies and pleasures as commodities, but the dynamics of a consumer-oriented economy had also packaged many products in sexual wrappings. *The commercialization of sex and the sexualization of commerce placed the weight of capitalist institutions on the side of a visible public presence for the erotic.* Political movements based on sexual issues alone, whether of the right or the left, faced huge obstacles in their efforts to alter the trend unless they tackled other issues as well. Sex was too deeply embedded in the fabric of economic life for a purity movement to reshape its meaning in fundamental ways. Exploitable as it was for profit, sex had become resistant to efforts at containment that failed to address this larger economic matrix. (p. 358, emphasis mine)

The sense of shame, were it not devalued and so non-chic in sophisticated circles, would certainly be a serious obstacle to modern capitalism's objectification of workers and consumers, its commercialization of sex, and its sexualization of commerce. Simply put, a strong resurgence of a healthy sense of shame would be bad for the economy. Hardest hit would be the publishing industry, the movie industry, the rock music industry, the television industry, the fashion industry, and the advertising industry, but business in general would suffer. *Time* magazine recently ran a cover story on what it called our foul-mouthed society, saying in effect "ain't it awful," but also saying that maybe some of this effluvia pouring forth from the mouths of various pop performers would be found to have true artistic value by some future generation. Hypocritically, we as a society fail to acknowledge the economic reasons for not cleaning up our act and pretend that it is only our great respect for the constitutional right of free speech and aversion to censorship that make us tolerate the rot eating away at the core of our culture.

THE CAMERA AND MODERN CONSCIOUSNESS

Samuel Coleridge defined a symbol as "part of the reality it represents." Thus, a historical event may symbolize the historical process of which it is a part. It is in that sense that Barfield (1977) sees the camera as a leading symbol of post-Renaissance man.

The camera and the vicissitudes of its development have so shaped our consciousness in unconscious ways that it is very difficult in these times to find a way of understanding the world uninfluenced by the camera. The camera, for instance, intensifies and reinforces the objective self-awareness originally bought about by the mirror and the objectifying gaze of the other that we discussed earlier. How impossible it would be to establish a modern-day ego without the photograph to make it clear that one is figure, outlined against the background of the world.

As D. H. Lawrence (1936b) put it,

We behave as if we had got to the bottom of the sack, and seen the Platonic Idea with our own eyes, in all its photo-

139

graphically developed perfection, lying at the bottom of the
sack of the universe. Our own ego!

The identifying of ourselves with the visual image of
ourselves has become an instinct; the habit is already old.
The picture of me, the me that is seen, is me. (p. 523)

Without this sense of oneself as that outlined figure in the
snapshot it would be very difficult indeed to provide the psychic
space in which a modern ego could really take hold. Many
people suppose that the ego, as currently understood, has been a
component of human personality throughout the last few mil-
lennia. I believe this view to be false and that the ego, as we know
it, is the result of the magnified objectification of the last few
centuries, which is closely tied to the camera and its precursors.

The camera has provided strong support for the notion that
the everyday world of our experience is an objective world
existing independently of any subject and thus has tacitly supported the objectivism that dominates modern science and philosophy. As Susan Sontag (1978) recognized, "The camera
makes reality atomic, manageable, and opaque" (p. 23). A photograph is accepted as an objective representation of some feature of the external world and is believed to have verisimilitude
superior to the subjective view of any individual observer. Never
mind that the photograph only has meaning to a subject. Sontag
observed that "photography implies that we know about the
world if we accept it as the camera records it. But this is the opposite of understanding which starts from *not* accepting the
world as it looks. All possibility of understanding is rooted in
the ability to say no. Strictly speaking, one never understands
anything from a photograph" (p. 23).

A consciousness based on the tacit metaphor of mind as
camera is a focused consciousness that frames a certain segment
of the world as deserving of special attention and by doing so
separates and isolates that segment from the rest of the world. It
denies continuity and interconnectedness. It is narrowly inclu-
sionary and broadly exclusionary. What is excluded from the
frame has no claim to existence in the world of photography or
in the consciousness shaped by the tacit camera metaphor. Cam-

140

era consciousness is the consciousness of science, which must frame, focus, isolate the field of study, record, and—in the process—ignore or derealize the larger world not included in the frame. As Susan Sontag (1978) noted: "In a world ruled by photographic images, all borders ('framing') seem arbitrary. Anything can be separated, can be made discontinuous, from anything else: all that is necessary is to frame the subject differently" (p. 22).

Camera consciousness also elevates a truncated form of visual experience over the other senses and thus disconnects and isolates sight from the other senses. We must remember, as Jonas (1974) points out, that sight isolated from other modes of experience is, in its essence, "superficial." Bound to the surface of things, it gives less information about the inner nature or condition of things than do the other senses. "It is the sense of appearances' par excellence, richest in their display, richest also in deception" (p. 227).

In Susan Sontag's book *On Photography*, which we have been citing, is a passage from Gustav Janouch's *Conversations with Kafka* that is germane to this discussion:

> In the spring of 1921, two automatic photographic machines recently invented abroad, were installed in Prague, which reproduced six or ten or more exposures of the same person on a single print.
>
> When I took such a series of photographs to Kafka I said light-heartedly: "For a couple of krone one can have oneself photographed from every angle. The apparatus is a mechanical Know-Thyself."
>
> "You mean to say, the Mistake-Thyself," said Kafka, with a faint smile.
>
> I protested: "What do you mean? The camera cannot lie."
>
> "Who told you that?" Kafka leaned his head toward his shoulder. "Photography concentrates one's eye on the superficial. For that reason it obscures the hidden life which glimmers through the outline of things like a play of light and shade. One can't catch that even with the sharpest lens. One has to grope for it by feeling. . . . This automatic camera doesn't multiply men's eyes but gives a fantastically simplified fly eye's view." (Janouch, cited in Sontag, 1978, p. 206)

Vision, in its broadest nonsuperficial sense, is more than *sight*; it is emotionally and intuitively informed seeing that penetrates mere appearance, integrates the other senses, the emotions, and the body as a whole. True vision depends on the eye of the heart. It is precisely this kind of vision of which the camera and camera consciousness are incapable.

The modern camera is the descendant of the camera obscura, which made its appearance in the 16th century. The camera obscura consisted of a darkened chamber with a small hole in one wall in which was fitted a small lens through which an image of the well-lighted external scene was projected onto the opposite wall of the darkened chamber. John Locke (1690/1952) clearly had the camera obscura in mind when he wrote the following in *An Essay Concerning Human Understanding*:

> I pretend not to teach, but to inquire; and therefore cannot but confess here again,—that external and internal sensation are the only passages I can find of knowledge to the understanding. These alone, as far as I can discover, are the windows by which light is let into this *dark room*. For, methinks, the understanding is not much unlike a closet wholly shut from light, with only some little openings left, to let in external visible resemblances, or ideas of things without: would the pictures coming into such a dark room but stay there, and lie so orderly as to be found upon occasion, it would very much resemble the understanding of a man, in reference to all objects of sight, and the ideas of them. (Book II, chap. XI, p. 147)

So, for Locke the mind becomes a camera obscura, and this way of conceiving of the mind became the guiding tacit metaphor for subsequent empiricists and is still very much a largely unconscious part of our 20th-century consciousness.

The magic lantern was born of experiments with the camera obscura and its modifications. The magic lantern was, of course, the name given to the earlier versions of what we know as the slide projector. Bailey (1986) in an essay entitled "Skull's Lantern" points to the enormous influence of the magic lantern on Western ways of thinking about mental processes. According to Bailey (and to Barfield, 1977, before him), this hidden collective image of the magic lantern metaphorically informed the way people began thinking about the functioning of the human mind, but the underlying metaphorical nature of the model was forgotten. Psychology began imagining the psyche projecting outward from a contained place, the skull. According to this view, when psyche is experienced outside this container, such experience must always be delusional, an error, and such experience must be withdrawn back inside. Bailey notes that "this delimitation of psyche's rightful place, however, distorts the very experience that it is intended to describe" (p. 73).

If psyche properly resides within the skull, as camera metaphors would lead one to believe, then it is an obvious and inevitable step to identify psyche with brain, as modern psychiatry and psychology have done. The idea that the mind is a function of the brain is not exactly a modern idea since Hippocrates viewed mental disorders as manifestations of brain abnormalities, but it's fair to assert that the currently almost unchallenged identification of mind with brain has been given additional grounding by tacit camera metaphors. Congress and the President, at the urging of the American Psychiatric Association and the National Institute of Mental Health, have declared the '90s the decade of the brain. NIMH officials and researchers are understandably excited about the prospect of obtaining ever-increasing moneys to fund their pet research projects, which will attempt to establish that all psychopathology is ultimately brain pathology. Unable to photograph the psyche, we perform an act of objectification and declare it isomorphic with the brain, which we can now examine more readily through the latest descendants of the camera, the various imaging machines that produce: CAT scans, MRIs, and PET scans. The phenomenal world according to neuroscience is the result of the final transformations of sense data somewhere in the brain. Yet the brain itself belongs to that phenomenal world. R. D. Laing (1976) asks, "How, as a member of the set we have to account for, can it be used to account for the set as a whole, and all members of the set, including itself?" (p. 22).

The camera and the mind-numbing onslaught of images made possible by still photography, motion pictures, and TV have led to the unrivaled supremacy of the visual as our favored mode of acquiring information about the world. When the visual apprehension of the world in Western culture becomes so magnified in importance and isolated from the body as a whole and its other sensory modalities, then it is inevitable that the issue of one's "image" also becomes greatly magnified in importance and isolated from one's grounding in a sense of community and a sensorially integrated self. "Image is everything," says tennis star Andre Agassi in a TV commercial for—guess what?—a camera, of course. The price one pays for living in a society dominated by the supremacy of the visual and being immersed in a sea of schlock images (on which floats the ship of capitalist economics) is that one's self seems to become more and more a matter of image. Politicians have understood, accepted, and exploited that trend more easily and readily than the rest of us; but it seems we are all apt to be nervous about our image—or if we are not, it is the mission of certain business interests, the advertising establishment, and the media to make us so.

One of the maxims of camera consciousness seems to be that anything that *can* be photographed *should* be photographed (and, at this point, presumably *has* been photographed by someone). Camera consciousness is thus opposed to a healthy sense of shame, which inhibits us from the temptation to objectify others. We are so far advanced in the cancerous process of camera thinking that we generally lack any clear awareness that to photograph others without their consent is in most cases an aggressive act (even *with* their consent it may be an aggressive act, as the photographs of Diane Arbus testify). To once again cite Sontag: "To photograph people is to violate them, by seeing them as they never see themselves, by having knowledge of them they can never have; it turns people into objects that can be symbolically possessed" (p. 14).

It is of related interest to note that when people are arrested and confined in jail perhaps the most important initial ceremonial act is the taking of "the mug shot." Nothing says "We've got you" quite like the mug shot; recall that when General Noriega was brought to the United States, every newspaper in the country had his mug shot on the front page.

Every day the TV camera invades another area of our life. We cannot go to the grocery store, shopping mall, bank, health club, major public building, or even the library without encountering the ubiquitous TV camera videotaping our transactions. We docilely accept this rampant objectification of ourselves on the grounds that it is a security measure. In recent years the TV camera has appeared in more and more legislative chambers and courtrooms, presumably to serve the public's "right to know" (a euphemism for morbid public voyeurism).

Daytime TV talk shows appear to earn their ratings on the basis of the sensationalistic insensitivity and tastelessness with which they relentlessly invade the ever shrinking boundaries of the private or personal. I believe it to be unfortunately true that such words as *crudeness*, *insensitivity*, and *tastelessness* have already become largely meaningless to great segments of the American population.

The following is a monologue by Jerome Stern, aired August 1, 1989, on "All Things Considered," National Public Radio's daily current affairs and news broadcast and subsequently published in *Harper's* (January, 1990):

I am watching *The New Newlywed Game*.
The host has just asked the wives to tell what their husbands will say when the husbands are asked what article of clothing is most likely to make them say, "Va va voom."
We already know how long they knew each other before they first made whoopee.
The couples joyfully betray each other for outdoor barbecue sets.
I think of them selling their most private acts, their personal intimacy, to the audience, which is laughing at their crossed stories and public squabbles.
"You don't remember that time in the kitchen?"
The audience whoops with salacious delight.
These people are clowns, with no sense of shame, no sense of privacy, of middle-class dignity.
I sink deeper into my depression at their eagerness to tell the world whether on their first date she was as slow as molasses or as easy as pie.
This is the ultimate in American tastelessness.
Then I begin to realize something.
These are not the people who have been fooled into believing that their lives are insulated by two-acre lawns and uniformed doormen.
The new newlyweds know that from elementary school on they've

145

been measured and quantified, that in order to get their jobs, what jobs they have, they have been credit-checked, back-ground-checked, and fore-ground-checked.

And they live lives of urine tests and blood tests and lie-detector tests and school transcripts and police records and intimate questionnaires and they have to give their social security numbers to anyone who asks them or go without what they want.

Every purchase they've ever charged, every blouse and jacket and motel bill, is on the computer. Their medication, their polyps, their bladders, their anxieties and depressions are all recorded as permanently as their dental X rays.

And should anyone believe they are of any significance, their neighbors will be questioned, their family investigated, and their old friends quizzed.

And the new newlyweds know this and manifest their lack of privacy with liveliness and vigor.

And their exhibitionism defies taste and dignity and redeems them.

The new newlyweds know they've been tagged, they've been bagged, they've been itemized, they've been inventoried, they've been weighed, they've been assayed, and they've been betrayed, and the only aspects of their lives that they control they control by saying them first.

What we give, you can't take.

These people are not fools,

For they understand the present and they foretell the future.

The new newlyweds act out our reality.

It is not a game. It is prophecy.

The only difference between us and you is that we're getting an outdoor barrbecue. (p. 27)

Stern's explanation for the readiness of the couples to betray one another in the revelation of aspects of their intimate life, although not without a measure of truth, seems to me insufficient. It isn't simply the fact that there are data of a quasi-personal nature (e.g., credit ratings, school transcripts, credit card purchase records, etc.) about all of us circulating through various information systems which constitutes the essence of what I call objectification. I don't feel personally negated or violated by being asked to disclose my social security number to someone, and I doubt that many people do (urine drug tests and blood tests are another matter). Objectification is more insidious and pernicious than that. Stern neglects the obvious point that the behavior he describes takes place in front of a camera. The camera deals with the realm of the explicit and the public. What is veiled cannot be photographed and therefore has no claim to respect as far as camera consciousness is concerned. The objectification associated with camera consciousness denies the legitimacy of the immediate, personal, or private. Since it is the persistent sense of shame that seeks to protect one's inner life and resists objectification, in a society dominated by objectifying camera consciousness the sense of shame has no legitimate place. In fact, it is a handicap to one's ability to adapt to such a society. Stern is right when he suggests that these couples on the *New Newlywed Game* "understand the present and foretell the future." Like Olympia, the stripper and starlet interviewed by Stoller (1979), they have chosen to embrace objecthood and be done with an interior life and with shame.

The primitive savage who feared the camera, believing it capable of stealing his spirit, understood something we haven't. According to Konig (1990):

> The "funny" belief of primitive tribes that being photographed would diminish them has been replaced by our equally "funny" belief that only through being photographed or filmed are we, our presence anywhere, our friends, our travels, made real. . . . In these brave new nineties we will be drowning in photo images. It is a reasonable guess that by the age of sixteen the average American or Japanese child of today has been photographed and filmed about as much as Charlie Chaplin. (p. 91)

We might as well include the French, Germans, and others as well. At a swimming pool in the south of France I recently watched a French couple, he with his camcorder, she with her 35-mm camera, faithfully record for at least 30 minutes every stroke and splash of their two young children as they tried to enjoy themselves in the water. I say "tried" because the incessant intrusion of the cameras and distraction of the parents calling to them, always trying for a better picture, must have made enjoyment difficult.

Konig suggests, and I agree, that we are addicted to images.

147

That addiction is fueled by an emptiness and boredom that only images can assuage. If "image is everything," as Agassi asserts, then being becomes nothing; and when being is nothing, boredom and emptiness are always at hand, threatening to envelop us. The only cure for boredom and emptiness is more images and so the circle is closed.

As D. H. Lawrence (1936a) wrote:

> If we could once get into our heads—or if we once dare admit to one another—that we are not the picture, and the picture is not what we are, then we might lay a new hold on life. For the picture is really the death, and certainly the neurosis, of us all. We have to live from the outside in, idolatrously. (p. 380)

SUMMARY

I have tried in this chapter to analyze the primary sources of the shamelessness that characterizes so many aspects of our society. Freud and subsequent psychoanalysts failed to respect the sense of shame and viewed it only as a neurotic affliction to be overcome. The enormous influence of Freudian ideas on the artistic community, the intelligentsia, and the educated public in the first half of this century made shamelessness, at least in sexual matters, the ideal of the enlightened liberal mentality. This disrespect for the sense of shame made it easy for capitalist institutions to commercialize sex and sexualize commerce. The third force contributing to our present state of affairs was the ever-increasing, demonic attraction of the photographic image and its emptying out of one's internal life in favor of one's image. As we saw in Chapter 4, concern with one's image is the essence of narcissism; if ours is a culture of narcissism, as Christopher Lasch (1978) dubbed it, then the camera has had a great deal to do with that.

·V·

Conclusion

A Last Word

The number of books on shame that have appeared in the last decade, books addressed to professional audiences as well to the general public, is evidence that the previously long-standing neglect of shame in the psychological and psychiatric literature has given way to a new awareness of the importance of understanding shame. I have attempted to show that certain widely held basic misunderstandings about shame were due in large part to the influence of psychoanalytic theory and practice on the mind-set of the educated public and on professionals in psychiatry and psychology.

As the reader has undoubtedly recognized, the theme that runs like a thread throughout this book is the connection between shame and objectifications of various kinds. I believe that this connection has been heretofore insufficiently appreciated; hence, the justification for a book of this kind.

The process of trying to gain a better understanding of shame, the most reflexive of all the affects, goes hand in hand with the process of gaining a better understanding of the nature of self experience. The ideas I have put forward are not easily assimilated into classical psychoanalytic theory or Kohution self psychology, but are probably more compatible with the latter.

Most of the recent literature on shame (Schneider, 1977, being a notable exception) has emphasized the negative aspects and usually failed to address the positive functions of shame or what I have referred to as the sense of shame. It's my hope that tha present work might help to restore a more balanced view of the role of shame in psychic life.

References

Amsterdam, B. (1972). Mirror self-image reactions before age two. *Developmental Psychobiology*, 5(4), 297–305.

Bailey, L. (1986). Skull's lantern. *Spring*, 72–87.

Balint, M. (1968). *The basic fault*. London: Tavistock.

Barfield, O. (1977). *The rediscovery of meaning and other essays*. Middletown, CT: Wesleyan University Press.

Barfield, O. (1985). *History in English Words*. Great Barrington: Lindisfarne Press.

Basch, F. (1983). Empathic understanding: A review of the concept and some theoretical considerations. *Journal of the American Psychoanalytic Association*, 31, 101–126.

Basch, F. (1988). *Understanding psychotherapy: The science behind the art*. New York: Basic Books.

Berger, J. (1977). *Ways of seeing*. New York: Penguin.

Bergman, I. (1970). *Bergman on Bergman* (interviews with Ingmar Bergman by Stig Bjorkman, Torston Manns, and Jonas Sima). New York: Simon & Schuster.

Broucek, F. (1977). The sense of self. *Bulletin of the Menninger Clinic*, 41(1), 85–90.

Broucek, F. (1979). Efficacy in infancy: A review of some experimental studies and their possible implications for clinical theory. *International Journal of Psychoanalysis*, 60, 311–316.

Broucek, F. (1982). Shame and its relationship to early narcissistic developments. *International Journal of Psychoanalysis*, 63, 369–378.

Buber, M. (1958). *I and Thou*. New York: Charles Scribner's Sons.

Bursten, R. (1973). Some narcissitic personality types. *International Journal of Psychoanalysis*, 54, 287–300.

Darwin, C. (1955). The expression of the emotions in man and animals. New York: Philosophical Library. (Original work published 1872)

Davidson, A. (1988). How to do the history of psychoanalysis: A reading of Freud's "Three essays on the theory of sexuality." In Meltzer (Ed.), *The trial(s) of psychoanalysis* (pp. 39–64). Chicago: University of Chicago Press.

D'Emilio, J., & Freedman, E. (1988). *Intimate matters: A history of sexuality in America.* New York: Harper & Row.

Emad, P. (1972). Max Scheler's phenomenology of shame. *Philosophy and Phenomenological Research, 32,* 361–370.

Erickson, E. (1950). *Childhood and society.* New York: W. W. Norton.

Farber, L. (1976). I'm Sorry Dear. In *Lying, Despair, Jealousy, Envy, Sex, Suicide, Drugs, and the Good Life.* New York: Basic Books.

Feldman, S. (1962). Blushing, fear of blushing and shame. *Journal of the American Psychoanalytic Association, 10,* 368–385.

Fenichel, O. (1945). *The psychoanalytic theory of neurosis.* New York: W. W. Norton.

Fossum, M., & Mason, M. (1986). *Facing shame: Families in recovery.* New York: W. W. Norton.

Freud, S. (1953). Three essays on the theory of sexuality. In J. Strachey (Ed. & Trans.), *The standard edition of the complete psychological works of Sigmund Freud* (Vol. 7, pp. 135–243). London: Hogarth Press. (Original work published 1905)

Freud, S. (1955). Group psychology and the analysis of the ego. In J. Strachey (Ed. & Trans.), *The standard edition of the complete psychological works of Sigmund Freud* (Vol. 18, pp. 69–143). London: Hogarth Press. (Original work published 1921)

Freud, S. (1957). On the history of the psychoanalytic movement. In J. Strachey (Ed. & Trans.), *The standard edition of the complete psychological works of Sigmund Freud* (Vol. 14, pp. 7–66). London: Hogarth Press. (Original work published 1914)

Freud, S. (1957). On the universal tendency to debasement in the sphere of love. In J. Strachey (Ed. & Trans.), *The standard edition of the complete psychological works of Sigmund Freud* (Vol. 11, pp. 177–190). London: Hogarth Press. (Original work published 1912)

Freud, S. (1957). On narcissism: An introduction. In J. Strachey (Ed. & Trans.), *The standard edition of the complete psychological works of Sigmund Freud* (Vol. 14, pp. 73–102). London: Hogarth Press. (Original work published 1914)

Freud, S. (1961). The ego and the id. In J. Strachey (Ed. & Trans.), *The standard edition of the complete psychological works of Sigmund Freud* (Vol. 19, pp. 12–66). London: Hogarth Press. (Original work published 1923)

Freud, S. (1961). Civiization and its discontents. In J. Strachey (Ed. & Trans.), *The standard edition of the complete psychological works of Sigmund Freud* (Vol. 21, pp. 64–145). London: Hogarth Press. (Original work published 1930)

Freud, S. (1963). Introductory lectures on psychoanalysis. In J. Strachey (Ed. & Trans.), *The standard edition of the complete psychological works of Sigmund Freud* (Vols. 15 & 16, pp. 9–496). London: Hogarth Press. (Original work published 1917)

Freud, S. (1964). New introductory lectures on psychoanalysis. In J. Strachey (Ed. & Trans.), *The standard edition of the complete psychological works of Sigmund Freud* (Vol. 22, pp. 5–182). London: Hogarth Press. (Original work published 1933)

Gabbard, G. (1989). Two subtypes of narcissistic personality disorder. *Bulletin of the Menninger Clinic,* 53(6), 527–532.

Gardner, J. (1978). *On moral fiction.* New York: Basic Books.

Gay, P. (1988). *Freud: A life for our time.* New York: W. W. Norton.

Glover, E. (1937). Contribution to the symposium on the theory of therapeutic results of psychoanalysis. *International Journal of Psychoanalysis,* 18, 125–132.

Greenson, R. (1967). *The technique and practice of psychoanalysis.* New York: International Universities Press.

Hermann, I. (1943). *Az emberiseg osi osztonei* [The primordial instincts of man]. Budapest: Pantheon.

Hillman, J. (1975). *Loose ends: Primary papers in archetypal psychology.* Dallas: Spring Publications.

Hillman, J. (1983). *Inter Views.* New York: Harper & Row.

Hillman, J. (1989). From mirror to window: Curing psychoanalysis of its narcissism. *Spring,* 49, 62–75.

Hoffer, E. (1974, October 18). Long live shame! *The New York Times.*

Izard, C. (1977). *Human emotions.* New York: Plenum Press.

Joffe, W., & Sandler, J. (1967). Some conceptual problems involved in the consideration of disorders of narcissism. *Journal of Child Psychotherapy,* 2(1), 56–66.

Johnson, M. (1987). *The body in the mind.* Chicago: University of Chicago Press.

Jonas, H. (1966). *The phenomenon of life.* Westport, CT: Greenwood Press.

Jonas, H. (1974). *Philosophical essays.* New York: Prentice-Hall.

Jones, E. (1953). *The life and work of Sigmund Freud.* (Vol. 1). London: Hogarth Press.

Kaufman, G. (1985). *Shame: The power of caring.* Cambridge, MA: Schenkman.

REFERENCES

Kaufman, G. (1989). *The psychology of shame*. New York: Springer.

Kernberg, O. (1975). *Borderline conditions and pathological narcissism*. New York: Jason Aronson.

Kinston, W. (1983). A theoretical context for shame. *International Journal of Psychoanalysis, 64*, 213–226

Kohut, H. (1971). *The analysis of the self*. New York: International Universities Press.

Kohut, H. (1977). *The restoration of the self*. New York: International Universities Press.

Konig, H. (1990, July). Notes on the mirror with a memory. *The Atlantic*, p. 91.

Kramer, P. (1990, September). *The Psychiatric Times*, p. 5.

Kunkel, F. (1931). *God helps those. . . .* New York: Ives Washburn.

Laing, R. (1976). *The facts of life*. New York: Pantheon.

Langs, R., & Stone, L. (1980). *The therapeutic experience and its setting*. New York: Jason Aronson.

Lasch, C. (1978). *The culture of narcissism*. New York: W. W. Norton.

Lawrence, D.H. (1936a). Book review of *The social basis of consciousness* by Trigant Burrow. In E. D. McDonald (Ed.), *Phoenix: The posthumous papers of D. H. Lawrence*. New York: Viking.

Lawrence, D. H. (1936b). Art and morality. In E. D. McDonald (Ed.), *Phoenix: The posthumous papers of D. H. Lawrence*. New York: Viking.

Levin, S. (1967). Some metapsychological considerations on the differentiation between shame and guilt. *International Journal of Psychoanalysis, 48*, 267–276.

Lewis, H. B. (1971). *Shame and guilt in neurosis*. New York: International Universities Press.

Lewis, H. B. (Ed.). (1987). *The role of shame in symptom formation*. Hillsdale, NJ: Erlbaum.

Lewis, H. B. (1988). The role of shame in symptom formation. In M. Clynes & J. Panksepp (Eds.), *Emotions and psychopathology*. New York: Plenum Press.

Lichtenberg, J. (1983). *Psychoanalysis and infant research*. Hillsdale, NJ: The Analytic Press.

Lichtenstein, H. (1963). The dilemma of human identity. *Journal of the American Psychoanalytic Association, 11*, 173–223.

Locke, J. (1952). An essay concerning human understanding. In R. M. Hutchins & M. Adler (Eds.), *Great books of the Western world*. Chicago: Encyclopedia Britannica. (Original work published 1690)

Lowenfeld, H. (1976). Notes on shamelessness. *Psychoanalytic Quarterly, 33,* 62–72.

Lynd, H. (1958). *On shame and the search for identity.* New York: Harcourt Brace Janovovich.

Malcolm, J. (1981). *Psychoanalysis: The impossible profession.* New York: Alfred A. Knopf.

Mannoni, O. (1982). *Ca n'empeche pas d'exister.* Paris: Seuil.

Margenau, H. (1984). *The miracle of existence.* Woodbridge, CT: Ox Bow Press.

Mayman, M. (1975, September). *The shame experience, the shame dynamic, and shame personalities in psychotherapy.* Paper presented to the Topeka Psychoanalytic Society. Topeka, KA.

Merleau-Ponty, M. (1964). *The primacy of perception.* Evanston: Northwestern University Press.

Miller, S. (1985). *The shame experience.* Hillsdale, NJ: The Analytic Press.

Miller, S. (1989). Shame as an impetus to the creation of conscience. *International Journal of Psychoanalysis, 70,* 231–243.

Morrison, A. (1983). Shame, ideal self, and narcissism. *Contemporary Psychoanalysis, 19,* 295–318.

Morrison, A. (1989). *Shame: The underside of narcissism.* Hillsdale, NJ: The Analytic Press.

Nathanson, D. (1987a). The shame/pride axis. In H. B. Lewis (Ed.), *The role of shame in symptom formation* (pp. 183–205). Hillsdale, NJ: Erlbaum.

Nathanson, D. (1987b). A timetable for shame. In D. L. Nathanson (Ed.), *The many faces of shame* (pp. 1–64). New York: Guilford Press.

Nunberg, H. (1955). *Principles of psychoanalysis.* New York: International Universities Press.

Papousek, H., & Papousek, M. (1975). Cognitive aspects of preverbal social interaction between human infants and adults. Ciba Foundation Symposium. In *Parent–infant Interaction.* New York: Association of Scientific Publishers.

Piers, G., & Singer, M. (1953). *Shame and guilt.* Springfield, IL: C. C. Thomas.

Plaut, E. (1990). Psychotherapy of performance anxiety. *Medical Problems of Performing Artists, 5*(1), 58–63.

Racker, H. (1968). *Transference and countertransference.* New York: International Universities Press.

Roustang, F. (1986). *Dire mastery.* Washington, DC: American Psychiatric Press.

Sardello, R. (1974). A phenomenological approach to development: The contributions of Maurice Merleau-Ponty. *Human Development, 17,* 401–423.

Sartre, J. P. (1956). *Being and nothingness.* New York: Washington Square Press.

Scheler, M. (1957). Uber Scham und Schamgefuhl. In Maria Scheler & M. S. Frings (Eds.), *Schriften aus dem nachlass. Gesammelte werke.* Berne: Francke Verlag. (Original work published 1913)

Scheler, M. (1970). *The nature of sympathy.* Hamden, CT: Archon Books. (Original work published 1912)

Schimek, J. (1987). Fact and fantasy in the seduction theory: A historical review. *Journal of the American Psychoanalytic Association, 35*(4), 937–965.

Schneider, C. (1977). *Shame, exposure and privacy.* Boston: Beacon Press.

Schuon, F. (1965). *Light on the ancient worlds.* London: Perennial.

Shapiro, D. (1989). *Psychotherapy of neurotic character.* New York: Basic Books.

Sharpless, E. (1985). Identity formation as reflected in the acquisition of person pronouns. *Journal of the American Psychoanalytic Association, 33,* 861–885.

Smith, W. (1984). *Cosmos and transcendence: Breaking through the barrier of scientistic belief.* La Salle, IL: Sherwood Sugden.

Sontag, S. (1978). *On photography.* New York: Delta.

Spiegal, L. (1966). Affects in relation to self and object. *The Psychoanalytic Study of the Child, 21,* 69–92.

Spitz, R. (1965). *The first year of life.* New York: International Universities Press.

Stern, D. (1983). Implications of infancy research for psychoanalytic theory and practice. In *Psychiatry Update* (Vol. 2). Washington, DC: American Psychiatric Press.

Stern, D. (1985). *The interpersonal world of the infant.* New York: Basic Books.

Stern, J. (1990, January). Newlyweds, newly considered. *Harpers,* p. 27.

Stoller, R. (1979). Centerfold: An essay on excitement. *Archives of General Psychiatry, 36,* 1019–1024.

Stoller, R. (1987). Pornography: daydreams to cure humiliation. In D. L. Nathanson (Ed.), *The many faces of shame* (pp. 292–307). New York: Guilford Press.

Straus, E. (1980). *Phenomenological psychology.* New York: Garland.

Szasz, T. (1963). The concept of transference. In R. Langs (Ed.),

Classics in psychoanalytic technique (pp. 25–36). New York: Jason Aronson. (Originally published in the *International Journal of Psychoanalysis, 44*, 432–443).

Thrane, G. (1979). Shame and the construction of the self. *The Annual of Psychoanalysis, 7*, 321–341.

Tinder, G. (1980). *Community: Reflections on a tragic ideal.* Baton Rouge: Louisiana State University Press.

Tomkins, S. (1962). *Affect, imagery, consciousness, Vol. 1: The positive affects.* New York: Springer.

Tomkins, S. (1963). *Affect, imagery, consciousness, Vol. 2: The negative affects.* New York: Springer.

Tomkins, S. (1981). The quest for primary motives: Biography and autobiography of an idea. *Journal of Personality and Social Psychology, 41*, 306–329.

Tomkins, S. (1987). Shame. In D. L. Nathanson (Ed.), *The many faces of shame* (pp. 133–161). New York: Guilford Press.

Trevarthen, C. (1974). Intersubjectivity and imitation in infants. *Bulletin of the British Psychological Society, 27*(95), 180–187.

Trevarthen, C. (1979). The tasks of consciousness: How could the brain do them? *Ciba Foundation Symposium, 69*, 187–215.

Tronick, E., Als, H., Adamson, L., Wise, S., & Brazelton, T. (1978). The infants response to entrapment between contradictory messages in face-to-face interaction. *Journal of Child Psychiatry, 17*, 1–13.

Wolfe, T. (1987). *The bonfire of the vanities.* New York: Farrar, Straus, Giroux.

Wurmser, L. (1981). *The mask of shame.* Baltimore: John Hopkins University Press.

Zaner, R. (1970). *The way of phenomenology.* New York: Pegasus.

Zaner, R. (1981). *The context of self.* Athens: Ohio University Press.

Index

Sexual drive/instinct
  Freud's theory, 108–115
  intrinsic regulation, 110
  Levin's views, 14
  psychophysiology, 115
  Scheler's formulation, 111–113
  sleep laboratory studies, 114
Sexual mores, 137
Sexuality, 105–119
  attitude toward, 136, 137
  commercialization of, 138, 139
  Freud's views, 108–115
  intrinsic regulation of, 110
  repression theory, 113, 114
  shame in the service of, 112–119
  shamelessness effects, 136, 137
Shame affect (*see* Affect system)
Shame anxiety, 39
Shamelessness, 130, 135–148
Shapiro, David, 79, 80
Shared consciousness, 33
Sight, 147
Sleep laboratory studies, 114
Social anxiety, 70
Social conformity, 18
Society and shamelessness, 135–148
Sontag, Susan, 140, 141
Splitting
  dissociative narcissism, 60–62
  versus secondary shame, 62
Stern, Jerome, 145–146
"Still-face" experiments, 31, 36
Stoller, Robert, 76, 122
Stranger anxiety, 31, 32
Straus, Erwin, 23, 24, 105
SUBJECT–object, 46–49
Subjective sense of self, 38
Superego, 113

"Switching on" experiments, 29
Szasz, Thomas, 87, 92

T

Television camera, 143–145
"Theatophilia," 14–16
Therapist
  interpretation problem, 98–102
  and objectification, 92, 101, 102
  objectivity myth, 84, 85
  rage toward, 88
  self-disclosure, 84, 85, 96
  in treatment situation, 83–102
"Three Essays on the Theory of Sexuality" (Freud), 11, 12, 108, 109
Tomkins, Silvan
  and early experience of shame, 30, 31
  narcissism theory, 60, 61
  and sexual inhibition theory, 112, 113
  sources of shame, 94, 95
  theory of shame, 20–22
Transference
  defensive function, 93
  humiliation relationship, 90–92
  and narcissism, 64
  and science, 87, 88
  shame in, 86–96
Trevarthen, Colwyn, 33, 34
Trust
  betrayal of, 107
  threat to, 19, 20
Turbulent narcissist, 61
TV camera, 143–145

V

Visibility, 23
Vision, 142
Voyeurism, 14, 15
  Freud's ideas, 105–107
  objectification, 137, 138
  role of shame, 105–107
  Straus's views, 23, 24

W

Western society, 130, 135–148
Women, 121, 134
Wurmser, Leon, 5, 14–16

Z

Zaner, Richard, 27, 32, 36